SYSTEMS FOR LARGE DATA BASES

2nd International IFIP Conference on
Very Large Data Bases
Brussels, Belgium, 8-10 September 1976

Sponsored by
International Federation for Information Processing, IFIP
and
ACM, (SIGIR, SIGMOD, SIGBDP)
IEEE Computer Society, (TC on Data Base Engineering)
Information Processing Society of Japan
DBMS Committee of Japan
US Army European Research Office
IBM World Trade (E/ME/A)

Program Committee

P. Lockemann (European Chairperson),
V. Y. Lum (American Chairperson),
M. Brockhaus, C, Delobel, G. G. Dodd,
L. Eswaran, J. S. Knowles, T. L. Kunii,
E. I. Lowenthal, H. Schappert, H. A. Schmid,
D. Tsichritzis, R. Yeh, C. A. Zehnder, D. W. Fife

NORTH-HOLLAND PUBLISHING COMPANY
AMSTERDAM • NEW YORK • OXFORD

# *SYSTEMS FOR LARGE DATA BASES*

Proceedings of the 2nd International Conference on Very Large Date Bases

edited by

P. C. LOCKEMANN
University of Karlsruhe
Karlsruhe, Germany

and

E. J. NEUHOLD
University of Stuttgart
Stuttgart, Germany

1977

NORTH-HOLLAND PUBLISHING COMPANY
AMSTERDAM • NEW YORK • OXFORD

North-Holland ISBN: 0 7204 0463 0

Published by:
NORTH-HOLLAND PUBLISHING COMPANY
AMSTERDAM • OXFORD • NEW YORK

Distributors for the U.S.A. and Canada:
Elsevier/North-Holland, Inc.
52 Vanderbilt Avenue
New York, N.Y. 10017

PRINTED IN THE NETHERLANDS

CONTENTS

## PREFACE

Because record-keeping and decision-making in industry and government are increasingly based on information stored in computer-processable data bases, the need for improved hardware and software technology for building, managing and using these data bases is becoming ever more important. This need is particularly acute in a complex society where the multitude and variety of interrelationships needs to be identified, represented, explored, explained and improved. The information covering these relationships that is necessary as basis for sound decisions grows more complex in nature and becomes more numerous in size. Furthermore, the increasing online use of computer systems and the emerging development of large-scale storage devices ($10^{12} \sim 10^{15}$ bits) suggests that a large share of future computer systems will be oriented towards the management of very large data bases.

The 2nd International Conference on Very Large Data Bases was held in Brussels Sept. 8 - 10, 1976, bringing together a wide range of data base experts from theoreticians through system designers to users, from the academic world through manufacturers to industrial and governmental applicants. The conference addressed itself to current issues and modern trends in the design implementation and use of management systems for data bases of up to several hundred million characters. This book contains the fifteen papers selected for the conference, covering subjects such as recent developments and trends in data base system architecture, approaches to the design of user languages and for supporting data models, techniques for performance improvements, communication and conversion of data between different data base management systems, and application support systems. The book documents some of the progress made in the field since the 1st International Conference on Very Large Data Bases took place in Framingham, Mass., Sept. 1975.

In selecting the papers to be presented at the conference, the program committee had the help of many wellknown specialists and we wish to thank all of them for their contributions.

We also want to thank the sponsors, supporters and cooperating societies who made this conference possible:

IFIP
ACM
  SIGIR
  SIGMOD
  SIGBDP
IEEE Computer Society
  TC on Data Base Engineering
Inf. Proc. Society of Japan
  Large Data Base Org. of Japan
University of Stuttgart
University of Karlsruhe
US Army European Research Office
Control Data Corporation
IBM Research Lab.
IBM World Trade (E/ME/A)

Conference Organization:

Conference Chairpersons:
Prof. E.J. Neuhold, Stuttgart, W-Germany (General Chairperson)
Dr. S.P. Ghosh, San Jose, USA (American Chairperson)
G.M. Nijssen, Brussels, Belgium (European Chairperson)

Program Committee:
Prof. P. Lockemann, Karlsruhe, W-Germany (European Chairperson)
Dr. V.Y. Lum, San Jose, USA (American Chairperson)
Prof. M. Brockhaus, Vienna, Austria
Prof. C. Delobel, Grenoble, France
Dr. G.G. Dodd, Warren, USA
Dr. K. Eswaran, San Jose, USA
Dr. J.S. Knowles, Aberdeen, Great Britain
Prof. T.L. Kunii, Tokyo, Japan
Dr. E.I. Lowenthal, Austin, USA
Dr. H. Schappert, Leverkusen, W-Germany
Dr. H.A. Schmid, Stuttgart, W-Germany
Prof. D. Tsichritzis, Toronto, Canada
Prof. R. Yeh, Austin, USA
Prof. C.A. Zehnder, Zurich, Switzerland
D.W. Fife, Washington D.C., USA

Local Organization Chairperson:
G.M. Nijssen, Brussels, Belgium

Treasurer:
H. Biller, Stuttgart, W-Germany

Registration Chairperson:
Ms. Maria Briers, Brussels, Belgium

Stuttgart, September 1976

Erich J. Neuhold

P.C. Lockemann

## Acknowledgements

Every paper submitted was carefully reviewed by four referees. Much of the reviewing was done by members of the Program Committee and the conference chairpersons, however, invaluable help was provided by the referees listed below.
Their assistance is gratefully acknowledged.

M. Astrahan
A. Bandurski
P. Bernstein
P.B. Berra
S. Braun
S. Brewer
C. Carlson
C. Chang
S.K. Chang
P. Chen
D. Chester
D. Choy
A. Dale
D. Dahm
R. Durchholz
E. Falkenberg
R. Frank
R. Gerritsen
G. Hanisch
F. Hossfeld
B. Housel
D. Hsiao
M. Huits
R. Kammüller
W.J. Kleefstra
K.D. Krägeloh
T. Lang
J. Lyon
C. Machgeels
F. Manola
E.J. McCauley
B. McGee
D. McLeod
G. Merten
J. Minker
F. Palermo
B. Plagman
J.G. Purdy
P. Raulefs
A. Reiter
E. Sacudati
J.L. Scott
M. Schkolnick
H.J. Schneider
J.R. Schroeder
S. Schuster
M. Senko
B. Shneiderman
E.H. Sibley
A. Smith
D. Smith
J. Smith
G. Stiege
S. Su
B. Taylor
E. Tozer
E. Vandijck
H. Visel
A. Wasserman
H. Wedekind
J.L. Weldon
S.B. Yao

*Systems for Large Data Bases, P.C. Lockemann and E.J. Neuhold, (eds.)*
*North-Holland Publishing Company, 1976*

# NEW CRITERIA FOR THE CONCEPTUAL MODEL*

W. Kent
IBM General Products Division
Palo Alto, California

In the three-level approach to data description, the conceptual or information level is supposed to provide a data independent model of the enterprise's information. It may be useful to examine the conceptual model in this light primarily, rather than as an extension of traditional data processing technology.

## THREE LEVELS OF DESCRIPTION

There is growing recognition of a need to provide and maintain three levels of data description ([ANSI], [GUIDE-SHARE]):

- o The multiple views held by a variety of applications, each employing their own variations on record formats, structures, and access techniques. This level is variously referred to as "application", "external", "program", and "logical".
- o The physical layout of data in storage, including implementation techniques for various paths and linkages. The common names for this level are "internal", "storage", and "physical".
- o The specification of the information content of the data base, employing concepts equivalent to entities, attributes, and relationships. Names for this level include "conceptual", "information", and "entity" (and, sometimes, "logical").

## RIGHT THE FIRST TIME?

The conceptual model will be a very real computer-related construct, just like a program or a data file. An enterprise is going to have a large amount of time, effort, and money invested in the conceptual model.

There is the learning investment. In spite of our best efforts, any formalism we adopt as the basis of the conceptual model will still be an artificial structure. The concepts will not be perfectly intuitive to anyone; the rules, limitations, and idiosyncrasies will have to be learned. There will be a formal language to be learned, as well as operating procedures. (Interactive facilities and other design aids may help -- after the bugs get ironed out -- but even their use has to be learned.)

Then comes the actual modelling effort. A lot of energy will go into forcing a fit between the model and the enterprise. The correspondences won't always be obvious; there will be lots of alternatives, and it will take some iterations to recognize the best choices. Sometimes it will take a flash of insight to perceive the real world in a new way, which better fits the model. Sometimes the enterprise itself will be altered to fit the model. (It's not unusual for a company to adopt a whole new part numbering scheme before automating their inventory control.) This is all accompanied by the gargantuan task of simply collecting and coordinating a mountainous heap of descriptions. "Many corporations will be carrying out the lengthy job over the next 10 years of defining the thousands of data-item types they use and constructing, step by step, suitable schemas from which their data bases will be built. The description of this large quantity of data will be an arduous task involving much argument between different interested parties. Eventually the massive data bases that develop will become one of the corporation's major assets" [Martin].

The end result will be a physically large volume of information. "It must be emphasized .... that the conceptual schema is a real and tangible item made most explicit in machine readable form, couched in some well defined and potentially standardizable language" [ANSI]. Think of it in the same orders of magnitude as a program library, or a system catalog, or a payroll file. Think of cylinders of disk space, and printouts many inches thick. Think of a small army of technical personnel who have been indoctrinated in a particular way of conceptualizing data, and who have mastered the intricacies of a new language and the attendant operational procedures.

All this time, manpower, and money will be invested by customers in the first conceptual model we really support in a major system. We had better be very careful about the architecture of that first one. Any attempt to replace it with a better one later will threaten that investment; customers won't accept the replacement any faster than they now accept a major new programming language, or a new operating system. And the replacements will forever be hamstrung by compatibility and migration requirements.

## THE LEGACY OF RECORD TECHNOLOGY

Records give us a very efficient basis for processing data. They enable us to map out very regular storage structures. They make it easy to write iterative programs for processing large volumes of data. They make it easy to partition data into convenient units for moving around, locking up, creating, destroying, etc.

In short, record technology reflects our attempt to find efficient ways to process data. It does not reflect the natural structure of information. Senko refers to "a major commitment to particular restrictive representations like the arrays of scientific computation, the extensional aspects of set notations, the n-tuples of relations, the cards, records, files, or data sets of commercial systems and the static categories of natural language grammars. Each of these representations has great merit for its original area of study, and in turn it has made major contributions to the study of information systems. Nonetheless, each provides only an approximate fit to the evolving, heterogeneous, interconnected information structures required to model real world enterprises" [Senko]. Sowa observes: "Historically, data base systems evolved as generalized access methods. They addressed the narrow issue of enabling independent programs to cooperate in accessing the same data. As a result, most data base systems emphasize the questions of how data may be stored or accessed, but they ignore the questions of what the data means to the people who use it or how it relates to the overall operations of a business enterprise" [Sowa 76].

Record technology is such an ingrained habit of thought that most of us fail to see the limitations it forces on us. It didn't matter much in the past, because our real business was record processing almost by definition. But we want to approach the conceptual model a little differently. We want it to reflect information, rather than data processing technology. When different applications deal with the same information using different record technologies, those differences shouldn't clutter up the conceptual model. (And we might want to consider the possibility of future data technologies which are not so record oriented.)

The legacy of record processing includes such traditions as these:

- Records preferably have a fixed number of fields.
- A record is an instance of one record type (perhaps implicitly, if there is only one record type in a file).
- The number of fields in the record is fixed for a given record type (a repeating pattern of fields is occasionally tolerated).
- The representation of each field is fixed for a given record type.
- One field (sometimes a combination of several fields) is designated as the key, whose values uniquely distinguish and identify occurrences of this type of record.
- As far as the system is concerned, a field name signifies a space in the record occupied by data in a certain representation. Any other semantic significance of the field name is perceived only by the user.
- The natural unit of data retrieval (and storage) is one of these records.
- Record formats are rigid and durable.

These are characteristics of a data processing technology. They are not the characteristics of entities and relationships. An entity can belong to many categories (unlike records and record types). Entities can have many names, and many kinds of names. They have multi-valued attributes. The information about them can be represented in many ways, and is often entangled with the information about other entities. And so on.

Traditions such as these don't die easily. They pervade <u>all</u> the major data models being seriously considered today. (I mean the IMS hierarchy, the DBTG network, the relational model, and even the ANSI proposal.) Mealy himself certainly encouraged the tradition by identifying entities with logical records. I think that the constraining influence of the record processing legacy should be seriously and objectively re-assessed before we commit ourselves to a particular structure for the conceptual model.

## Representation of Relationships

The record oriented approach fosters an asymmetry in the treatment of relationships. One-to-many relationships are given fundamentally different treatment from many-to-many relationships. [Martin] refers to many-to-many relationships as "complex plex structures", and says "The reason for making the distinction between simple and complex plex structures is that the latter need more elaborate methods for representing them physically."

This treatment arises from the traditional aversion to repeating fields in a record, and from the convenience of lumping two things into the same record when there happens to be a singular relationship between them.

An m:n relationship, such as the one between employees and skills, cannot be represented in either an employee record or a skills record without repeating fields (e.g., a skills record containing a list of the employees having that skill). For that reason, m:n relationships are accorded the status of an independent entity by introducing a third record type ("intersection record") to represent it. Each record of this type represents the association between one skill and one employee. The record will also (correctly) contain any attributes relevant to that relationship, such as the amount of experience the employee has in that skill. The relationship is thus represented as a distinct piece of information, its attributes are clearly identifiable, and it is even named (the name of the record type, or relation).

The 1:n relationship between departments and employees could be represented as a list of employees in a department record, but no record processing technologist would be so foolish. However, a single department number fits very comfortably into an employee record, so the relationship is traditionally lumped into the same record which carries so much other information about the employee. This relationship is not treated as an independent entity, because there is no implementational motivation to do so.

Furthermore, singular (non-repeating) attributes of the relationship also tend to get lumped into that same record (e.g., date of transfer into department). Thus a record may contain the attributes of an entity, some of the relationships which that entity has with other entities, and attributes of those relationships. This may make sense in a pragmatic record processing environment, but is it an appropriate way to model entities and relationships in a conceptual model?

People are quick to defend intersection records on the grounds that (1) the relationship is symmetrically a fact about both entities involved, and (2) attributes of that relationship may exist separately from attributes of the related entities. Strangely enough, these arguments are always advanced on behalf of m:n relationships, and never for 1:n relationships. The relationship between an employee and a department is as much a fact about the department as about the employee. People are reluctant to acknowledge this in employee records, but proclaim it vigorously in employment history records, where the relationship happens to be m:n.

The record oriented tradition imposes biases into the conceptual model which have nothing to do with the information content of the data base. The biases reflect the preferred practices, limited capabilities, and performance constraints of today's data processing technology.

One application may wish to see a department number in an employee record, while another may wish to see a list of employees within a department record. For one application, a department record should include the current manager's date of assignment; for another, that fact belongs in the manager's personnel records. These alternatives reflect different ways of perceiving and using the information, not differences in the information itself. Record oriented models force a bias in these alternatives; in each case one of the alternatives must be chosen, thereby creating a preference.

Suppose that one did specify in a conceptual model that the employee record contains the department number. I would guess that any real system would then disallow:

- Storing the information as lists of employees within departments, even if that is eventually found to give the best performance tradeoffs for the installation.

- Materializing employee lists within department records for an application. The ANSI proposal suggests that this can be supported by introducing the second format into the conceptual model, along with some correspondence specifications. Why should the conceptual model be cluttered so, when no new information is being added?

## Naming Relationships

A relationship could have as many as three names associated with it -- one for each direction, plus a "neutral" one. The relationship between parts and warehouses might be called:

- "Inventory". This might occur as the name of the file, (intersection) record type, relation, segment type, etc. which represents the relationship.

- "Stored in". This might occur as a role name associated with the warehouse domain.

- "Contains". This might occur as a role name associated with the parts domain.

An ideal system should probably recognize the three kinds of names (and three corresponding syntaxes) for the relationship.

There is no systematic way to specify or detect a relationship name in most current systems and models. The neutral type of name is only likely to occur when the relationship is m:n, because of its implementation in a distinct record type which needs to be named. The directed names might not occur at all in an m:n relationship (the field names in the inventory file might simply name the domains --

parts and warehouses). Except, that is, when the domains are the same; then both directed names are employed as role names to distinguish them ("assembly" and "component" in a parts explosion relationship).

If the relationship is 1:n, then sometimes no relation names will occur (consider the field named "dept" in an employee record), and sometimes the name associated with the many-to-one direction will occur as a role name (e.g., if someone had thought to name that field "employed in dept").

In any case, the hunt for a relationship name is hampered by the usual lack of any formalism for separating the role and domain components of a field name.

The DBTG facility for naming relationships also reveals similar inconsistencies. Set names name 1:n relationships. For an m:n relationship, the name is a record type (the intersection record). In addition, there still exists the conventional capability of representing a relationship by a data item in a record [Nijssen 75].

## Several Concepts of "Domain"

Record technology also leads to a confusion between data items and the information they represent. This shows up in certain interpretations of the domain concept.

The main uses of the domain concept are to:

- o Provide a means of indicating what sorts of values are meaningful or acceptable for a given attribute. Equivalently, a domain defines which entities may participate in an explicitly declared relatonship.
- o Indicate when a relationship might be inferred on the basis of common attributes. (E.g., if a supplier and a warehouse both have an attribute in the domain of cities, then a certain relationship between the supplier and the warehouse may be inferred.)

These two uses lead to two somewhat different domain concepts, which tend to get confused. In the second usage, a domain may be viewed as an entity type, e.g., employees or dates, regardless of how the entities are named or represented.

The alternate view is to treat a domain as a set of data items, or data objects, which then becomes entangled with choices of names and representations. This view is very common, occurring, e.g., in [ANSI], [Hammer], and [Eswaran]. In this view, people's names, employee numbers, and social security numbers each comprise a separate domain (any of which might be used to identify employees). Similarly, Julian dates, month/day/year, day/month/year (and the variations of these representing months as numbers, abbreviations, or full spellings) might each be considered a separate domain. Sometimes there is an attempt to classify these domains as either strings or numbers [Hammer], although I haven't explored how or why the distinction is made. (Various kinds of computations might be performed on the various representations of date; some of these representations appear to be more "numeric" than others.)

This second sense of domain may be appropriate for a manipulative interface or for implementation structures, but not for classifying entities in the conceptual model. For the conceptual model, it should be sufficient to specify that an employee's manager comes from the domain of employees; there is no need to involve the domain of employee numbers. An integrity rule should be specified as "an employee may not be his own manager"; there is no need to specify whether employee names or numbers should be compared (as proposed, e.g., in [Hammer] and [Eswaran]).

The two concepts of domain might be reconciled by specifying a domain as a family of related representations, with conversion procedures provided among them ([Eswaran], [ANSI]).

Even this approach admits of varying degrees of success in approximating a true entity concept. Most trivially, such a domain might be defined over all numeric data types, with appropriate conversion routines provided. All numeric data would then be considered to be in the same domain -- hardly an entity concept.

The next level of sophistication might associate domains with concepts of measure. Length, area, volume, time, money, etc., might each be defined as a domain, again with conversion routines provided within the domain. Here again, we might ask whether all things measurable by length are the same type of entity.

More progress: define separate domains for things with common units of measure, but which aren't really comparable entities. [Eswaran] illustrates this by distinguishing the domains for an employee's height and his distance from work.

There is a spectrum of sophistication here, moving from data items to the concept of an abstract thing which might be represented by any member of an "equivalence class" of data items. However, the only proposal I have seen which carries the concept far enough is in [Hall]. The tendency has been to limit such equivalence classes to things which can be numerically computed from each other (data types, units of measure). Consider two situations:

- Determine whether a certain order was received on the same date a certain person was hired (allowing dates to be represented differently in the two places).

- Determine whether any employees are also stockholders (allowing people to be represented by employee numbers in one place and social security numbers in the other).

The tendency is to say that in the first case we may compare directly on dates, and the system will provide automatic conversions to obtain a common represenation. The same facility is not extended to the second case; the user cannot compare on the common domain of "people", but must instead navigate through a third relationship which matches employee numbers with social security numbers.

For the conceptual model, we should have a concept of "domain" which makes a better separation between entities or values and their representations in data items. [Hall] makes the same proposal.

## SEMIOTICS

The relevance of semiotics (a branch of philosophy dealing with the theory of signs) to data processing has been stressed by such authors as Zemanek and Stamper. It is a natural connection, since a computer deals only with the signs which represent things, and not with the things themselves.

Some authors equate signs with information, defining semiotics as "the theory of information (or of signs and signals)", and then further defining information as "the output of a mapping process, in the form of analog or digital signs or signals" [Tully].

This approach is tempting because it deals with quantifiable, measurable things. It lends itself to manageable theories, testable hypotheses, probability theorems, and other impresssive mathematical paraphernalia. It lets one compute how many redundant bits have to be sent down a noisy channel to achieve a certain probability of correct reception at the other end. (It doesn't ask what those bits might mean to anybody.)

It is a powerful ally to the approach to information which is founded on records and data items. It's the same philosophy.

This interpretation of semiotics is the wrong approach for the conceptual model. As its name implies, the conceptual model should describe concepts, not signals. Signals and concepts correspond very poorly. The argument is much the same as the earlier disussion of domains. To illustrate: I consider a person's weight to be a single piece of information. Depending on the units and precision of measurement, this information can have many representations. Since each representation comprises a different "sign" or "signal", a narrow semiotic approach to information would treat each representation as a distinct piece of information. What is needed here is a concept of "equivalence classes" of signals which all convey the same meaning. Information as a concept would then correspond to these equivalence classes themselves, rather than to the signals comprising the classes.

Conversely, such a narrow approach to information would fail to deal with the fundamental problem of ambiguity, wherein the same signal may convey different meanings in different circumstances. In general, we might have a many to many relationship between signals and concepts.

Tully himself unwittingly encounters the duality between information as signs and as concepts when he says "<u>information</u> is a mapping or model of something else (which could be an object, or an event, or some other <u>information</u>)" (my emphasis).

Computers do deal only in signs; a data base is only a collection of signs. From these premises one can easily -- and incorrectly -- conclude that the conceptual model describes a collection of signs.

The models themselves are ensembles of signs; and in particular the signs designate <u>sets</u> of things (the external and internal models contain signs describing sets of records and fields, not individual instances). The external and internal models are appropriately constrained to describe sets of signs, since what is being described there consists of things which can be processed by programs and stored in devices.

But the conceptual model need not suffer this restriction. There is no reason why we can't introduce signs naming sets of <u>things</u> ("employees", "departments") distinct from signs for the sets of signs which name such things ("employee numbers", "social security numbers", "department codes", "department names").

In the conceptual model, we make assertions about members of sets. By distinguishing sets of things from sets of signs, we can avoid confusing several kinds of assertions:

- Assertions about real things: "every employee must be assigned to exactly one department".
- Assertions about signs: "a department code consists of a letter followed by two numbers".
- Assertions relating things and signs: "a department has exactly one department code and one department name".

With such separations, we can more clearly approach a semantic bridge to reality in the conceptual model, by explicitly relating sets of signs to sets of things.

## FUTURE MODELS

It may be too late to advocate new directions, because the effort to adopt and standardize structures for descriptive models is already well under way ([ANSI], [DBTG]). This is unfortunate, because I don't think a good structure has been fully developed as yet.

The popular models of today are driven by computer technology. This is appropriate for the external model, which must be primarily concerned with effective and efficient algorithms for processing data; and for the internal model, whose primary concern is to provide efficient storage structures and access paths. These two interfaces are expected to reflect computer technology, and to be responsive to advances in the technology. "Information systems technology has relied solely on fact representations which arose from card and tape media. These representations will have continued utility both at the user interfaces for human efficiency in transaction specification and at the interface to physical media for computer efficiency, but to provide further improvements in data independence we will probably have to supplement them with a compatible, more neutral form of fact representation at the system interface. We may gain clues about the form of this supplement from the freer form work on mathematics and linguistics" [Senko].

What has not yet been generally realized is that the criteria for a good conceptual model may be quite different from the criteria at the other levels. The priorities are reversed: the conceptual model is <u>primarily</u> a model of the information used in the enterprise. "The creation and maintenance of the conceptual data base schema is considered to be a business operations responsibility rather than an information systems operations responsibility and, administratively, would report to or be part of the enterprise's operations organization" [Bachman]. The model is just barely constrained by computer technology; there always does have to be a reasonable way to map from the conceptual model to the external and internal models.

But the conceptual model wants to be minimally impacted by changes in computer technology.

My intuition suggests that the right model will:

- o Have a generalized graph structure.
- o Have entities and relationships as primitive constructs.
- o Allow entities to belong to many categories.
- o Not confuse entities with their names and representations.
- o Not display anything readily recognizable as a record.

There is a significant amount of work heading in this direction, such as the "idea structures" of Griffith. Graph structures almost invariably emerge when the primary objective is the representation of information, rather than data processing ([Bell], [Bobrow], [Heidorn], [Schank], [Shapiro]). Various efforts to provide a semantic layer around the relational model have led to graph structures ([Sowa], [Roussopoulos], [Schmid], [Sharman]).

[Bernstein] makes a subtle shift in the view of the relational model by treating functional dependences as the primitives from which relations can be derived. This is a step toward treating named relationships as primitive concepts. It is only a partial step, since functional dependences do not identify m:n relationships, and they are not named, or accessible as a part of the data.

This all adds up to a very significant trend in the theory of information representation. It would be unwise to ignore it.

## REFERENCES

[Abrial] J.R. Abrial, "Data Semantics", in [Klimbie].

[ANSI] ANSI/X3/SPARC, Study Group on Data Base Management Systems, Interim Report, Feb. 1975. Also in FDT (Bulletin of ACM SIGMOD) 7 (2), 1975.

[Bachman] C.W. Bachman, "Trends in Database Management - 1975", National Computer Conference, 1975.

[Bell] A. Bell and M.R. Quillian, "Capturing Concepts in a Semantic Net", Proc. Symp. on Associative Information Techniques, Sept. 30-Oct. 1, 1968, Warren, Mich., pp. 3-25.

[Bernstein] P.A. Bernstein, J.R. Swenson, and D.C. Tsichritzis, "A Unified Approach to Functional Dependencies and Relations", in [SIGMOD 75], pp. 237-245.

[Bobrow] D.G. Bobrow and A. Collins (ed.), Representation and Understanding, Academic Press, 1975.

[Chen] P.P.S. Chen, "The Entity-Relationship Model: Toward a Unified View of Data", ACM Transactions on Database Systems 1 (1), March 1976, pp. 9-36.

[CODASYL 71] CODASYL Data Base Task Group Report, ACM, New York, April 1971.

[DBTG] Same as [CODASYL 71].

[Eswaran] K.P. Eswaran and D.D. Chamberlin, "Functional Specifications of a Subsystem for Database Integrity", in [VLDB 75], pp. 48-68. Also IBM Research Report RJ1601.

[Griffith 73] R.L. Griffith and V.G. Hargan, "Theory of Idea Structures", IBM Technical Report TR02.559, April 1973.

[Griffith 75] R.L. Griffith, "Information Structures", IBM Technical Report TR03.013.

[GUIDE-SHARE] "Data Base Management System Requirements", Joint Guide-Share Data Base Requirements Group, Nov. 1970.

[Hall] P.A.V. Hall, J. Owlett and S.J.P. Todd, "Relations and Entities", in [Nijssen 76].

[Hammer] M.M. Hammer and D.J. McLeod, "Semantic Integrity in a Relational Data Base System", in [VLDB 75], pp. 25-47.

[Heidorn] G.E. Heidorn, "Natural Language Inputs to a Simulation Programming System", Report NPS-55HD72101A, Naval Postgraduate School, Monterey, 1972.

[Klimbie] J.W. Klimbie and K.L. Koffeman (eds.), _Data Base Management_, North Holland, 1974.

[Martin] J. Martin, _Computer Data-Base Organization_, Prentice-Hall, 1975.

[Mealy] G.H. Mealy, "Another Look at Data", Proc. AFIPS 1967 Aug. 28, 1975, pp. 365-370.

[Mumford] E. Mumford and H. Sackman (eds.), _Human Choice and Computers_, North Holland, 1975.

[Nijssen 75] G.M. Nijssen, "Two Major Flaws in the CODASYL DDL 1973 and Proposed Corrections", Information Systems, Vol. 1, 1975, pp. 115-132.

[Nijssen 76] G.M. Nijssen (ed.), _Modelling in Data Base Management Systems_, North Holland, 1976.

[Roussopoulos] N. Roussopoulos and J. Mylopoulus, "Using Semantic Networks for Data Base Management", in [VLDB 75], pp. 144-172.

[Schank] R.C. Schank and K.M. Colby, _Computer Models of Thought and Language_, W.H. Freeman, 1973.

[Schmid] H.A. Schmid and J.R. Swenson, "On the Semantics of the Relational Model", in [SIGMOD 75], pp. 211-223.

[Senko] M.E. Senko, "Information Systems: Records, Relations, Sets, Entities, and Things", Information Systems 1 (1), 1975, pp. 1-13.

[Shapiro] S.C. Shapiro, "The Mind System. A Data Structure for Semantic Information Processing", Rand Corp., Santa Monica, California, Aug. 1971.

[Sharman] G.C.H. Sharman, "A New Model of Relational Data Base and High Level Languages", Technical Report TR.12.136, IBM United Kingdom, Feb. 1975.

[SIGMOD 75] ACM SIGMOD International Conference on Management of Data, May 14-16, 1975, San Jose, California, W.F. King (ed.).

[Sowa 76] J.F. Sowa, "Conceptual Graphs for a Data Base Interface", IBM J. Res. & Dev. 20 (4), July 1976, pp. 336-357.

[Sowa] J.F. Sowa, Conceptual Structures: Information Processing in Mind and Machine, Addison-Wesley, forthcoming.

[Stamper 73] R. Stamper, Information in Business and Administrative Systems, John Wiley, 1973.

[Stamper 75] R. Stamper, "Information Science for Systems Analysis", in [Mumford].

[Tully] C.J. Tully, "The Unsolved Problem -- A New Look At Computer Science", Computer Bulletin 2 (2), Dec. 1974.

[VLDB 75] Proceedings of the International Conference on Very Large Data Bases, Sept. 22-24, 1975, Framingham, Mass. (ACM, New York)

[Zemanek] "The Human Being and the Automaton", in [Mumford].

*Systems for Large Data Bases, P.C. Lockemann and E.J. Neuhold, (eds.)*
*North-Holland Publishing Company, 1976*

# STRUCTURE AND REDUNDANCY IN THE CONCEPTUAL SCHEMA IN THE ADMINISTRATION OF VERY LARGE DATA BASES

Herbert S. Meltzer
International Business Machines Corporation
San Jose, California

This presentation explains the role of the conceptual schema in securing management control over very large data bases and in providing data independence for users of the data. The conceptual schema can also be used to describe the information model of an enterprise. The conceptual schema is presented as a tool of data base administration.

This presentation addresses structure and redundancy in the conceptual schema. Two philosophies exist concerning permissible mappings between an external schema and the conceptual schema. One, to provide maximum derivability of information from the data, assumes an unstructured, non-redundant conceptual schema, third normal conceptual record sets, and permits arbitrarily structured external records to be defined in terms of combinations of conceptual records. The other, to provide dynamic data independence during attribute migration and control over the information that can be derived from the data, assumes a highly structured, highly redundant conceptual schema, third normal,...,unnormalized conceptual record sets, and requires external records to be subsets of predefined conceptual records. A complete data base management system should provide both capabilities, and enforce constraints when each may be used.

## 1. INTRODUCTION

It is gratifying to find almost universal acceptance of what was once considered by many to be a highly controversial set of objectives and a very speculative architecture -- as proposed in the 1971 report of the joint GUIDE-SHARE Data Base Management System Requirements Group[1]. It is gratifying technically, because this signals the beginning of a data base technology generation capable of coping with an environment of very large data bases undergoing continual evolution and change. It is gratifying personally, because of the contributions to this technology of my 1969 presentations to GUIDE and SHARE[2], proposing this architecture to satisfy these objectives.

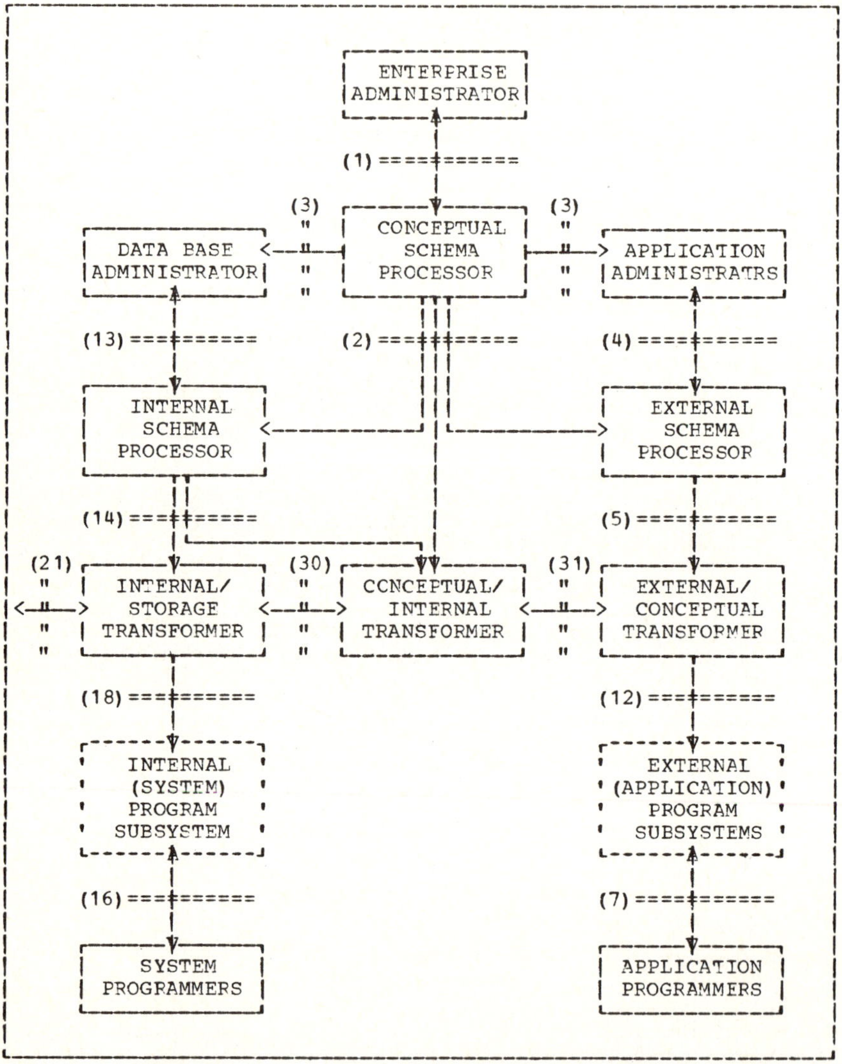


FIGURE 1. SIMPLIFIED SYSTEM SCHEMATIC.

It is well understood and accepted that a three-level architecture (stored, entity, logical of GUIDE-SHARE[1]; internal, conceptual, external of ANSI SPARC[3]; contrast with the two-level architecture, subschema, schema of CODASYL Data Base Task Group[4]) is useful to provide static data independence and is necessary to provide dynamic data independence.

However, there is controversy over the place of structure and redundancy in the conceptual schema, and in permissible transformations between objects defined in the conceptual schema and objects defined in an external schema.

Figure 1 shows a simplified system schematic developed by ANSI SPARC embodying a three-level architecture. Not shown in Figure 1, but implied in the architecture, are interfaces (languages) to describe the potentially complex transformations performed by the transformers of objects defined in each of the schemata to corresponding objects defined in other schemata. The transformation algorithms cannot always be deduced simply from inspection of the source and target descriptors. The phrase "mapping between schemata" means defining the algorithms for these transformations.

This presentation assumes familiarity with the requirements for management control over the content, use and eventual disposition of the data in a highly integrated, highly shared data base; and for data independence[1 2 3 5]. This presentation will examine the phenomena of dynamic data independence and of attribute migration, and how particular properties of the conceptual schema and of the binding and mapping languages best assist data base administration to cope with these problems.

## 2. BINDING AND MAPPING OF OBJECTS TO EACH OTHER

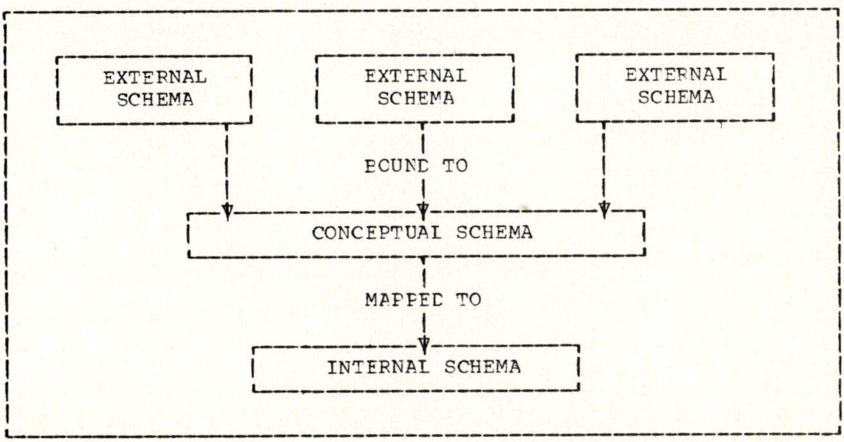


FIGURE 2. BINDING AND MAPPING OF OBJECTS TO EACH OTHER.

The conceptual schema is one of three sets of descriptors used to describe and control a data base. Figure 2 shows the three schemata and their interconnections. The external schema contains descriptors of the external record sets, external records and external fields as seen by and manipulated by users and application programs. The conceptual schema contains descriptors of the conceptual record sets, conceptual records and conceptual fields that constitute an information model of an enterprise. The internal schema contains the descriptors of the internal record sets, internal records and internal fields as they are maintained in the data base. A data base is completely described by one internal schema specifying how the data is actually stored, one conceptual schema specifying what data may be retained and how that data may be viewed and manipulated by different users and applications (thus providing control over the contents and usage of the data) and as many external schemata as necessary to subset and tailor a view for a user or family of applications. The conceptual schema is mapped to the internal schema, and each external schema is bound to that portion of the conceptual schema to which it corresponds.

The enterprise administrator writes the conceptual schema. An application administrator, analyst, or programmer writes an external schema and binds the objects declared in his external schema to objects declared in the conceptual schema. Data name binding is a function usually provided in an operating system control language. The data base administrator writes the internal schema and the mappings of objects declared in the conceptual schema to objects declared in the internal schema.

A mapping can be as simple as one-to-one name association for objects that are structured congruently; or it may be quite complex for an object that is constructed of parts of several other objects, for an object that is virtual, or for an object that is stored redundantly to enhance recoverability or response time. Dynamic mappings, which change from form extent to form extent, are even more complex to write.

The degree of complexity is limited, first by the flexibility of the data base management system, and then by the economic constraints of the use of that data -- the greater the constraint on response time, the simpler the mappings have to be, the less freedom different users have in viewing the same data different ways, and the less the capability of the data base administrator in retuning the data base without expensive conversions.

Please distinguish between the logical structure of the external data, as materialized in an external record set, the apparent structure of the conceptual data, as described in a conceptual record set, and the physical organization of the internal data, as stored in an internal record set. Any of these may be relational, hierarchic, network (or any other ingeneous construct already invented or yet to be invented). The relative simplicity, clarity, meaningfulness of any of these to a user has been amply discussed elsewhere. This discussion is neutral to all of these. In a flexible implementation, different structures and organizations could coexist. It will be shown that all are useful concurrently in defining a conceptual schema. Please also distinguish between all of these and the hierachic construct of bindings and mappings advocated in this paper. Finally, please distinguish between redundancy of data in storage, and redundancy of definitions in the conceptual schema. The value of redundancy of data in storage is economic -- cost of storage and cost of maintenence of consistency versus ability to recover and speed of retrieval. The value of redundancy of definitions in the conceptual schema is the thesis of this paper. In a flexible implementation, redundancy in definition and redundancy in storage are individually controllable.

## 3. STRUCTURE AND REDUNDANCY IN THE CONCEPTUAL SCHEMA

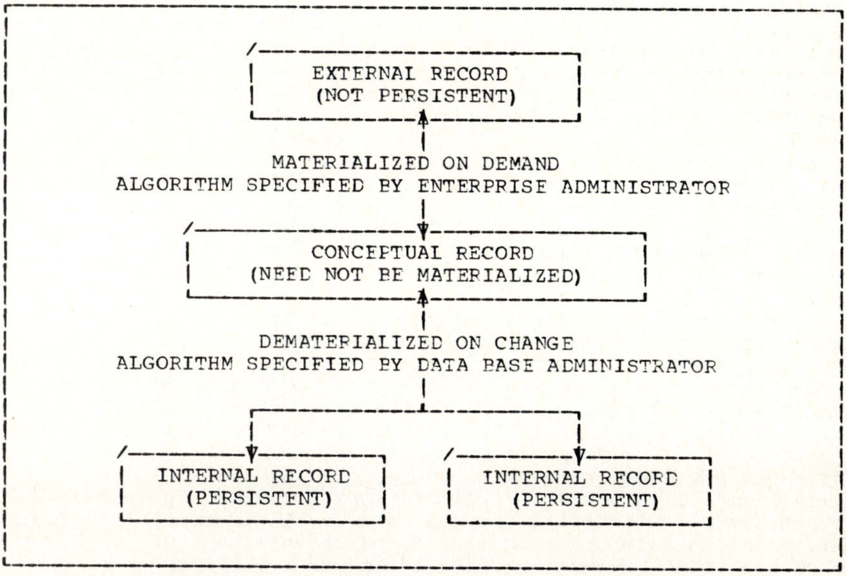


FIGURE 3. MATERIALIZATION OF RECORDS.

Two philosophies exist concerning structure and redundancy in the conceptual schema and the permissible mappings between an external schema and the conceptual schema. More precisely, the permissible operations that can be specified for the transformation of all or parts of one or more objects defined in the conceptual schema to an object defined in an external schema. Still more precisely, the permissible operations that can be specified by an application administrator, to augment the algorithm prespecified by the data base administrator, for the transformation of all or parts of one or more stored objects defined in the internal schema to an application's object defined in an external schema -- assuming objects defined in the conceptual schema need not be materialized as an intermediate step in this transformation. The path of materialization is shown in Figure 3.

One philosophy envisions that the conceptual schema consists of (essentially non-redundant) descriptors of elementary conceptual objects, most usefully in third normal form. The external-to-conceptual mapping language enables creation of external descriptors of complex, highly structured objects from selection and combinatorial operations upon conceptual descriptors of simple objects. That is, an external record can be a construct of one or more conceptual records. This has the advantage that there is no limit to the external objects that can be defined in terms of conceptual objects; and there is no mathematical constraint to appropriate operations on conceptual objects. This permits maximum derivability of information from the data.

The other philosophy envisions that the conceptual schema consists of (essentially highly redundant) descriptors of complex, highly structured objects. The external-to-conceptual binding language enables identification of and association with the conceptual descriptors of which the external descriptor is a nested subset. That is, an external record set must be a subset of the conceptual record set to which it is bound, and an external record must be a subset of the corresponding conceptual record. There are one or more predefined conceptual record set descriptors for each external record set descriptor (more than one if a given application can operate upon different bodies of similar data, e.g., different months of sales data, and thus a given application's external record sets can be bound to different conceptual record sets). This has the advantage of simpler binding language, and of tighter control by by the enterprise administrator over the structures that may be viewed by an application.

There is no technological argument in favor of one compared to the other. Either is equally easy or hard to implement -- a complex mapping language and sophisticated transformer must be developed whether the mapping be above or below the conceptual schema. Both have the same performance implications -- an object materialized from parts of other objects takes just as long to materialize whether the mapping be above or below the conceptual schema. The performance difference depends upon the degree of data independence: if the materialization algorithm must be interpretive to preserve data independence, it's going to be slow; if a compiler may a priori resolve the descriptors from the stored object to the application's object at the expense of data independence, it can be faster. The argument is operational: a highly redundant, highly structured conceptual schema provides the user dynamic data independence even during attribute migration, and provides the enterprise administrator stronger controls.

Please distinguish between value to a (non DP) user of structure as perceived in an external record set, and value to a data base administrator using structure in the conceptual schema to control and grow the data base.

The problems usually associated with redundancy -- e.g., maintaining consistency among multiple copies, more complex (bifurcating) locking paths, increased storage requirements -- are due to redundancy in the internal model, and not to redundancy in the conceptual model. Redundancy in the conceptual model increases the number of logical paths to a stored object, thus increasing the difficulty of recognizing interference, but this is the same kind of problem as multiple physical paths to an object (e.g., network internal schema). Redundancy in the conceptual schema can grossly inflate the data dictionary mechanism, aggravating an already significant problem in very large, highly shared data bases; the enterprise administrator can balance the human factors tradeoff between thumbing through a huge collection of conceptual record descriptions to find one suitable for the application and thumbing through a smaller collection forced to select among conceptual record descriptions none of which is obviously suitable (i.e., precisely tailored) for the application.

The conclusion is obvious -- for research or browsing type applications over appropriate portions of the data, and for bread and butter type applications over more controlled portions of the data -- a complete data base management system should provide both capabilities, and control over who may use each over what portion of the data. However, in my opinion, if it be necessary to simplify the design, then ability to control is of higher priority than ability to browse.

## 4. DYNAMIC DATA INDEPENDENCE

Data independence is a capability of a data base management system that insulates a program's use of stored data from interference of other programs and from the trauma of evolution of the data environment and of the technology.

Static data independence is the ability to cope with change in the "everyone out of the pool" mode. All processing of that body of stored data is stopped. All the descriptors are rewritten. All the stored data is converted (possibly automatically) to correspond to the new descriptors. All the programs that access the stored data are converted (possibly automatically) to correspond to the new descriptors. When this conversion is complete for the entire data base, then processing can resume.

A two-level descriptor system can be sufficient to provide static data independence. There are now several widely used systems that provide static data independence.

Dynamic data independence is the ability to cope with change when there are not two stable states, the pre-existing and the target, nor the ability to suspend processing during the conversion. Dynamic change can be characterized as the concurrent existence of different form extents of representation, organization, indexing, access paths, materialization algorithms, for the same kind of data. Some examples of dynamic change are:

- A real time system often can't be taken down while the stored data is reconfigured and reorganized.
- All stored records containing employee pay data written before January 1 have four digit local tax fields, while all stored records written after January 1 have five digit local tax fields.
- Regulations may require that certain fields be expunged from existing stored records. This can be done incrementally, over the time allowed by those regulations, without disrupting all other use of the same stored records during the conversion.
- In some systems different priorities and response requirements exist on different portions of the same stored data, requiring the stored data to be partially reorganized -- more frequently, incrementally reorganized.
- Stored records may take different forms as they age. All stored records that are over three months old have quarter-to-date figures actually in them. In newer stored records, because the numbers are still changing, these figures are computed by the system each time the record is

read. When a stored record ages three months, that figure is actually inserted. The program need not know whether the data is actually stored, or is materialized on demand.

The data base management system dynamically provides the data to the user or the user's program as it expects to see the data. Therefore, the stored data need not be completely converted, and the programs need not be recompiled, for the processing of the stored data to proceed. Binding of the characteristics of the data as required by the applications to the characteristics of the stored data is at command execution time for dynamic data independence. If interpretive processing is necessary to enforce fine-grained selective security, or to ensure validity and consistency of stored data, then the incremental cost of dynamic data independence may be low.

Dynamic variation therefore has two aspects: (1) the existence of different form extents of the same kind of stored data with different sets of descriptors, and (2) the possibility of "rolling conversion" concurrent with processing. In the former situation, the mixture of different formats may coexist for an extended period of time, with all of the old stored records remaining in the earlier format, and all the new stored records conforming to the new format. In the latter situation, the conversion mechanism shares the data base (in contention) with concurrent applications, and applications can utilize stored data subject to time-variable descriptors, with the system insulating them from the time variability.

CONCEPTUAL RECORDS BEFORE ATTRIBUTE MIGRATION:

| WIDGET | GREEN | 3.1 |
|---|---|---|

| JONES | SCHOOL | WIDGET | 95 | 68 | 3.98 |
|---|---|---|---|---|---|

EXTERNAL RECORD BEFORE ATTRIBUTE MIGRATION:

| JONES | SCHOOL | WIDGET | 95 | 3.98 |
|---|---|---|---|---|

FIGURE 4. OBJECTS DEFINED BEFORE ATTRIBUTE MIGRATION.

Another characterization of data independence involves the dynamics of changes to views with respect to changes to stored data. If applications' views can change and evolve while the storage organization and configuration must be held constant, then that can be called static. If both the applications' views can change and evolve, and the storage organization and configuration can change and evolve concurrently, and neither will hold still so a single generation of maps can be drawn from one to the other, then that can be called dynamic. It is necessary for some set of descriptors to hold still, so that each of the sets that vary can be mapped to a stable intermediate.

Dynamic data independence permits more of an evolutionary process of coping with change, rather than a one-time concentrated revolutionary process. A two-level descriptor system cannot provide dynamic data independence; it is required that there be a three-level descriptor system.

## 5. ATTRIBUTE MIGRATION

One aspect of data independence that is not widely appreciated is coping with a semantic change to the enterprise's information model. This change is known as attribute migration. An example of how evolution of business practices cause attribute migration involves pricing. At one time, prices were negotiated with each subcontractor for each product for each project on which it is used. As shown in Figure 4, the record type that had the combination of fields "SUBCONTRACTOR, PROJECT, PRODUCT" as the identifier was the one that included the field "PRICE."

CONCEPTUAL RECORDS AFTER ATTRIBUTE MIGRATION:

| WIDGET | GREEN | 3.1 | 3.98 |
|---|---|---|---|

| JONES | SCHOOL | WIDGET | 95 | 68 |
|---|---|---|---|---|

| JONES | SCHOOL | WIDGET | 95 | 68 | 3.98 |
|---|---|---|---|---|---|

EXTERNAL RECORD AFTER ATTRIBUTE MIGRATION:

| JONES | SCHOOL | WIDGET | 95 | 3.98 |
|---|---|---|---|---|

FIGURE 5. OBJECTS DEFINED AFTER ATTRIBUTE MIGRATION.

Later, business practices changed to set a uniform price for each product. Then the record type that had the combination of fields "SUBCONTRACTOR, PROJECT, PRODUCT" as the identifier was no longer the one that included the field "PRICE," but, as shown in Figure 5, the record type that had the field "PRODUCT" as the identifier became the one that included the field "PRICE." This phenomenon of a field being moved from one record type to another is an example of attribute migration. As a matter of fact, pricing practices may be different for different products at the same time. Thus, attribute migration can occur in space as well as time.

This is a change to the conceptual schema, the information model. Whether there should be a corresponding change to the internal schema, the storage model, is a separate, economic consideration.

Some applications may be sensitive to this change. Other applications that need prices, but are not sensitive to how they are negotiated, should not be impacted by these changes in the enterprise, nor by their reflection in the data base. The sensitive applications must have the external records redefined, and have the definitions bound to the new conceptual record definitions. The non-sensitive applications can retain the external record definition, and can retain the binding to the redundant conceptual record definition.

By defining redundant conceptual record sets in the conceptual schema, the enterprise administrator can preserve applications' views to cope with attribute migration, to preserve stability, and to provide data independence.

Let me emphasize -- the conceptual schema is not really stable, because it must reflect real changes in an environment that is continually and uncontrollably changing. Because the conceptual schema can be redundant, it can retain prior definitions, and can appear stable to applications that need not be impacted by these changes.

## 6. MANAGEMENT CONTROL OVER VIEWS OF DATA

The responsibilities and functions of data base administration are well documented[6] [7] - - -. One function, preservation of data security, involves control over access to data. More precisely, control over the derivation of information from access to the data base.

It is possible for an application to derive information from structure of data, as well as from values of data. A collection of data may be defined with essential structure. If certain values are secured from the application (e.g., salary) but corresponding structure is not (e.g., sequence by salary), then security may have failed. This example is oversimplified and trivial to be obvious.

To assist the enterprise administrator in controlling access to structure as well as values, each conceptual record set definition can specify both the structure and contents of the corresponding collection of data. The same collection of data otherwise structured would constitute a different conceptual record set with a different name. The same collection of data in third normal form would constitue still another (more likely more that one other) entity record set. Subset collections, or superset of subset collections would constitue still other entity record sets. Thus the same collection of data could appear redundantly in different conceptual record sets.

By requiring external record sets to be subsets of conceptual record sets, external records to be subsets of conceptual records, and by controlling the conceptual record sets to which an application can bind its external record sets, the enterprise administrator can control both the values and the structure to which that application has access.

## 7. EFFECT OF STRUCTURE AND REDUNDANCY IN THE CONCEPTUAL SCHEMA

Very large data bases are most often found in environments of integration, growth and change; unanticipatable by, uncontrollable by, and unmanageable by data base administration. In fact it is such growth and integration that build very large data bases, and alter the relative values and priorities of the applications that operate upon them. Therefore, very large data bases are very prone to evolution in unanticipated directions, both in application and configuration, and to sharing among applications unknown to each other. Very large data bases are especially susceptible to requirements for response and performance that require tuning and retuning.

Omitting the conceptual schema from the binding path, and binding the names and characteristics of objects described in an external schema (objects known to an application) directly to the names and properties of objects described in the internal schema (objects as they are actually stored) has a specific and predictable effect reducing data independence and management control.

If all applications are designed to work only on specific, predeterminate, bodies of stored data, and if all the characteristics of these bodies of stored data are always uniform and known in advance, then a two-level system of schemata and static binding, e.g., by a compiler, can be satisfactory. Allocation of functions and timing are not technical issues. The placement of the conceptual schema in the binding path between an external schema and the internal schema is useful to static data independence. It permits a data base administrator to write m + n instead of m x n mappings and generations of mappings.

However, if any application is designed to work generically (on alternate, substitutable, bodies of stored data), or if any of the characteristics of these bodies of stored data may be varied between reprocessings (recompilations), or may be non-uniform over the body of stored data (form extents), then a three-level system of schemata and the capability for dynamic binding (i.e., during execution) are required. This capability is technically very sensitive to the allocation of functions and timing among the processors and schemata. The placement of the conceptual schema in the binding path between an external schema and the internal schema is essential to provide the level of indirection essential to dynamic data independence.

To accommodate parameterized, generic applications it is necessary to provide a function similar to operating systems control statements to name the conceptual record sets to which that application's external record sets are to be bound for that execution.

To accommodate concurrent changes in application's views and in storage organization, it is necessary for the conceptual schema to hold still, so that each of the schemata that vary can be mapped to that stable intermediate. To me, it is less important that the conceptual schema contains a conceptual overview of the enterprise's information than that the conceptual schema can appear to remain stable, permitting the internal schema and the external schemata to evolve decoupled from each other.

To accommodate evolving application's views and attribute migration, it is necessary to permit these views to be preserved in the conceptual schema. That is, the conceptual schema contains different conceptual record and conceptual record set descriptors, which describe the same data in different associations and structures. Thus, the descriptors are redundant -- whether the stored data is redundant depends upon other performance considerations and tradeoffs. Obviously, these different descriptors of the same data have different names. If an attribute migrates from one conceptual record to another, new descriptors are added to the conceptual schema; and the former descriptors are retained redundantly, if applications bound to them can still run properly. An application's external record sets and external records are bound to the conceptual record sets and conceptual records that display the associations and structures the application requires.

This is how structure and redundancy in the conceptual schema accommodates attribute migration and preserves stability during evolution of the business.

By defining conceptual record sets, authorization to use them, and requiring that external record sets be subsets of conceptual record sets, the enterprise administrator can control applications' views of data. By augmenting the conceptual schema, he can support additional views, and he can integrate into the data base the evolution of the enterprise's information structure.

This is how structure and redundancy in the conceptual schema provides the enterprise administrator stronger controls.

By rewriting the internal schema, the data base administrator can cause the data base management system to retune the data base. By rewriting or augmenting the mappings between the internal schema and the conceptual schema, he can alter the algorithms used by the data base management system to materialize applications' data, thus providing data independence.

This is how the conceptual schema is used to accomplish these data base administration tasks: establishment of a more global view of the information in the enterprise, control over content, control over usage, control over sharing, and protection of investment in programs and stored data.

REFERENCES

1. Data Base Management System Requirements, Joint GUIDE-SHARE Data Base Management System Requirements Group, November 11, 1970. Available from GUIDE International, c/o Smith, Bucklin and Associates, Inc., 111 East Wacker Drive, Chicago, IL 60607.

2. Herbert S. Meltzer, Data Base Concepts and Architecture for Data Base Systems, Presented to SHARE Information Systems Research Project, August 20, 1969. Available from IBM Corp., 5600 Cottle Road, San Jose, CA 95193.

3. Interim Report, ANSI/X3/SPARC Study Group on Data Base Management Systems, 75-02-08. Available from Computers and Business Equipment Manufacturers Association, 1828 L Street NW, Washington, DC 20036.

4. CODASYL (Conference on Data Systems Languages) Data Base Task Group Report, April 1971. Available from Association for Computing Machinery, 1173 Avenue of the Americas, New York, NY 10026.

5. Herbert S. Meltzer, Current Concepts in Data Base Design, Presented at the Association for Systems Management International Systems Meeting, May 15, 1973. Available from IBM Corp., 5600 Cottle Road, San Jose, CA 95193.

6. The Data Base Administrator, GUIDE Data Base Administration Project, April 16, 1973. Available from GUIDE International, c/o Smith, Bucklin and Associates, Inc., 111 East Wacker Drive, Chicago, IL 60607.

7. Establishment of a Data Base Administration Function, SHARE Data Base Project, June 4, 1974. Available from SHARE Inc., Suite 750, 25 Broadway, New York, NY 10004.

*Systems for Large Data Bases, P.C. Lockemann and E.J. Neuhold, (eds.)*
*North-Holland Publishing Company, 1976*

# A SEMANTIC MODEL FOR DATA BASE PROTECTION LANGUAGES*

H. Rex Hartson
The Department of Computer Science
Virginia Polytechnic Institute and State University
Blacksburg, Virginia 24061
Phone: (703) 951-5232

and

David K. Hsiao
The Department of Computer and Information Science
The Ohio State University
Columbus, Ohio 43210

KEYWORDS

security space model, protection languages, protection, security, data security, access control, data base systems, semantic model, access conditions, protection requirements, authorization, enforcement, validation

ABSTRACT

The authorization process in a protection system is the process which translates and stores specifications of all protection requirements. In giving recognition to the authorization process, this work develops a model of access control to provide a semantic base for constructs of protection languages at many levels of sophistication, accommodating a wide range of protection policies. The concepts of "authorizer" and "ownership" are used for validation of authorizations in the model. The basic sets of the model are presented. Subsets of states are defined by restrictions on resource values, described by Boolean expressions known as conditions. The most important use of conditions is as access conditions, which allow each access decision to depend on information related to the user, to resources, to data content, to access history, and to the general state of the system. A GENERAL class of users is defined to establish an overall minimum level of access rights without an explicit representation for each and every user. The enforcement process is described and illustrated by an example.

## SCOPE

The need for access control is well motivated in the literature. The purview of this work is limited to logical access control and does not include administrative aspects, physical access control, or cryptography. It also does not deal with the profound implications of "information protection" [BAUMR75, HANSM71], which involves inference of the semantics of data contents. It also assumes an effective

---

*The work reported herein is supported by the Office of Naval Research, through contract NØØØ14-75-C-Ø573. This paper is based largely on a part of the first author's Ph.D. dissertation [HARTH75].

solution to the problem of user identification and that there is no "back door" or "sneak entrance" through which any user can surreptitiously by-pass the protection processes. Economic considerations are not a primary part of these results, but they were taken into account throughout the development. Furthermore, the work concentrates on protection in a data base environment.

## 1. MOTIVATION OF APPROACH

A protection system has both an authorization process and an enforcement process. Protection requirements are presented to the authorization process. Subsequently, access requests are presented to the enforcement process which, by consulting the protection requirements, renders an access decision. Models exist for protection mechanisms [SALTJ75]. However, existing models of protection almost universally emphasize the enforcement process to the exclusion of the authorization process. This paper gives recognition to the authorization process. As an immediate result, the concept of protection languages, the means by which access control information of all kinds can be entered into protection systems, is introduced. Protection languages are intended to replace the typically crude present methods for entering access control information, allowing the use of a broader spectrum of authorization policies.

A protection language construct is a semantic entity associated with a particular protection feature or function. This paper presents a model of protection to be used as a semantic foundation for the constructs in a family of protection languages in much the same sense that Dennis' common base language model provides a base for the fundamental constructs of programming languages [DENNJ72].

Consideration of authorization also draws several other concepts into the model. For example, the "authorizer" emerges as an entity distinct from the "user". Authority can now be decentralized, if desired, from the bottleneck of a single data base administrator. Also the concept of ownership acquires a role more general than its traditional one [DENNJ66, BARRD67, HSIAD68], and the concept of validation of protection specifications becomes an explicit part of the model.

The view of protection through authorization and protection languages points out a deficiency in current models of protection. The access matrix [LAMPB71, GRAHG72] (a common model of access control information) and its variations represent access rights as a function of three variables: user, resource, and operation. Yet, many protection requirements call for access decisions to depend on quite a number of other things [HOFFL69, FRIET7Ø, CONWR72, BRAND73]. The concept of an access condition is introduced to accommodate these broader dependencies.

This study also brings the issue of policies versus mechanisms into sharper focus. Policies are broad, externally defined tasks to be accomplished by users of the computing system. On the other hand, a mechanism is a set of primitive functions with which implementations of policies can be built. Although this distinction is well understood at the level of program instruction sets and machine architecture, it is often ignored at the system level. A notable exception to this neglect is the work on HYDRA, described in [JONEA73, WULFW74]. Application of this principle in the security space model lends much of the motivation for its broad generality, allowing many decisions typically built into protection mechanisms to be realized as higher policy decisions.

## 2. CONCEPTS AND TERMINOLOGY

### 2.1 OWNERSHIP

That a user is the owner of a particular data unit usually means he created the data or he entered the data into the system. The important implication is that he has the legal authority to grant access privileges (with respect to that data) to other users. He also has the authority to share his ownership with other users. This ownership authority is not necessarily the exclusive property of a system administrator (SYSADMIN) nor is it necessarily a permanent privilege of any individual in the system. The SYSADMIN is usually declared to be the sole owner of certain system resources. In most systems the SYSADMIN has certain administrative responsibilities requiring access privileges beyond those of the average user. The extent of the SYSADMIN's power, however, is a question of policy.

Ownership may also be determined dynamically. Under the conditions which determine a user to be an owner of a data unit, he may grant access rights to that data unit. Under other conditions, he may not.

## 2.2 SETS OF THE MODEL

Several sets are involved in the conceptual model of access control for language constructs. The model is based on sets of n-tuples (n-ary relations) over these sets. These basic sets are introduced in this section.

### USERS

An important set of the model is the set of individual users, $\underline{U}$, who will be making access requests. Sets of users will be called user groups.

### AUTHORIZERS

There is also a set of individuals who will be granting authorizations, the authorizers, $\underline{A}$. An authorizer is the owner of data units and has the responsibility of making authorizations, i.e., of determining who may share in the access of those data units and in what manner. In the literature the term "user" is almost universally used to denote both users of the data base system and users of the protection system. The distinction is emphasized here by using the term "authorizer" because of its importance in the authorization process.

### RESOURCES (DATA)

The collection of all data elements forms the set of resources. A data element is the smallest entity which can be accessed or named on an individual basis. The terms "data element" and "resource" are equivalent.

Since this model is not tied to a particular model of data, the nature of a data element depends on the resolution of data definitions in a given application. A data element may correspond to, for example, a single field of a record in a file or to a single attribute within a tuple of a relation. Subsets of data elements will be referred to as data units.

All accessible physical resources, such as tape drives, channels, disk controllers, and even CPU registers, are represented to the system via an address and/or logical name plus, sometimes, status indicators and other values associated with the operation of the devices. Therefore, these physical resources are viewed as part of the data. Since the model is oriented toward a database environment, the term data will commonly be used to refer to this set. To mnemonically emphasize the inclusion of all resources the name $\underline{R}$ is used for the set.

ELEMENTAL DATA OPERATIONS

The operations a user may perform on the data elements also comprise a set, $\underline{E}$. Examples of operations are: OPEN, CREATE, READ, WRITE, ADD, UPDATE, DELETE, EXECUTE, COMPARE, DISPLAY, OWN, and SUBOWN.

NOTATION

The following notation will be used. Underscored upper case letters will denote sets while lower case letters, possibly subscripted, will denote set elements. Finally, subsets will be denoted by upper case letters, possibly subscripted. Subscripts will follow the associated variable, delineated by square brackets when necessary for clarity. For example, s, s[1], or s1 is an element of S, while S = {s[1], s[2]}={s1,s2} is a subset of $\underline{S}$ = {s[1],s[2],s[3]} = {s1,s2,s3}.

Various structures may be imposed upon these sets, if desired. For example, experience may incline one to impose hierarchical structures on the users, the data elements, or the data operations. Those structures certainly can be accommodated, but they will not be assumed, and nothing in this work will depend on such assumptions. These structures represent policies, not fundamental mechanisms. As such, they should not be built into a basic model of protection nor, many times, immutably fixed in a given implementation.

2.3 SYSTEM STATES AND CONDITIONS

RESOURCE VALUES

In dealing with the set of data elements, the content or values of the data elements are of particular interest. The data elements in $\underline{R}$ may be enumerated as follows: r1,r2,...,r[n]. Let $\underline{V}$(r[i]) denote the set of all possible values for data element r[i]. All possible contents of the data base system (all possible combinations of values)are characterized by the cartesian product:

$$\underline{S} = \bigtimes_{i=1}^{n} \underline{V}(r[i])$$

The product, $\underline{S}$, is the set of all states in the data base system; i.e., $\underline{S}$ is the set of all possible combinations of values over all data elements. There are now five basic sets in the security space model--namely, $\underline{U}$, $\underline{A}$, $\underline{R}$, $\underline{E}$, and $\underline{S}$.

A single state of the data base system may be represented by an n-tuple as follows:

(v(r1), v(r2),...,(v(r[n])),

where v(r[i]) $\varepsilon$ $\underline{V}$(r[i]), for i=1,2,...,n. That is, a state corresponds to one combination of one value for each data element.

CONDITIONS

The use of all possible values in the expression for $\underline{S}$ corresponds to the set of all system states. State subsets are defined by placing restrictions on the values of some of the data elements. A practical means for specifying these restrictions is a predicate, called a condition, which partitions the set of all states into two equivalence classes: those for which the predicate is true and those for which it is false. Such a predicate will generally be in the form of a logical combination of comparison expressions.

Some examples of comparison expressions are:

$\underline{alpha} \leq 7.56$

$\underline{x} = \underline{y}$

$(\underline{r1} + 3752) > (\underline{pi} * (\underline{r2})**2)$

Herein is adopted the convention from programming languages that, in an expression, a data name, r[i], actually refers to its value, v(r[i]). Further, data names will be in lower case and underscored, and character string values will be in single quotes. Expressions may also include values other than purely numeric ones (e.g., character strings, sets, and relations, trees, lists).

In conditions, comparison expressions may be connected by ∧ (AND), ∨ (OR), and ¬ (NOT). An example of a predicate containing the above comparison expression is:

$(\underline{alpha} \leq 7.56) \wedge ((\underline{x} = \underline{y}) \vee ((\underline{r1} + 3752) > (\underline{pi} * (\underline{r2})**2)))$

Although conditions have been defined as descriptions of sets of states, conditions can also be used for testing membership of other kinds of sets. Let C(b,B) be a condition associated with a set B. Membership of B is dependent on C(b,B) in the following way:

$$B = \{b:C(b,B) \text{ holds}\}$$

A condition is said to hold if, upon evaluation, it has a value of "true". In other words, a candidate b is a member of set B if and only if C(b,B) holds for b. And, since the truth value of C(b,B) is in general varying with time (with database system state), membership of b in B is a dynamic property. The element b is an unconditional (non-)member of B if C(b,B) has a constant value of "true" ("false"). To determine if a candidate b is an element of B, the logical expression for C(b,B) is evaluated and then the above set definition for B is applied.

If the set in question is U, a group of users, then C(u,U) determines whether or not an individual user u has membership in user group U at a specific instant in time and C(u,U) is called a <u>user group defining condition</u>. Similarly, C(r,R), where r is a data element and R is a data unit, is called a <u>data unit defining condition</u>. An important use of a condition is as an <u>access condition</u>, C(s,S), which defines the set of states for which a given type of access is allowed.

The reader should understand that the original definition of "condition" (in terms of states) is still the one being used throughout.

Recall that a condition is a description of a range of data values and a state is a single "snapshot" of all the data values at a given instant in time. Therefore, each condition, no matter what its use, always defines a <u>set</u> of states. A user group defining condition, however, defines a set of users as well as a set of states. The set of states defined by C(u,U1), for example, contains just those states of the database for which a candidate user, u, is to be considered a member of U1. The two sets are related by an isomorphism, and it is generally more convenient to think only of the set of users. Since all user identification information is part of the database and therefore contributes to the system state, there is no conflict between the two viewpoints.

Within the model there are no restrictions on what type of variables can be used in any of the conditions. However, it is reasonable to restrict each condition type to certain classes of variable types in a specific implementation.

## USER GROUP DEFINING CONDITIONS

A user group can be defined by a list of user identifiers. The examples in this section illustrate a second way—the use of conditions to define user groups. The simplest of these definitions is the one for a standing group called GENERAL. Its defining condition is:

C(u,GENERAL) = "true"

Thus, every user is implicitly and unconditionally a member of the GENERAL group, sharing its minimum level of privileges. This is an answer to the problem of wasting storage to represent, for example, the rights of everyone to use a public file [LAMPB71].

The following are typical of the user group defining conditions which can be dynamically evaluated.

$$C(u,U1) : \underline{dept}(u)=13 \vee \underline{project}(u)='design'$$

$$C(u,U2) : \underline{classcode}(u)='ab.x' \wedge \underline{orgn}(u)='acm'$$

$$C(u,U3) : \underline{term1}(u)=42$$

$$C(u,U4) : \underline{subsys}(u)='fortran'$$

When a user logs in, if he is either in department 13 or part of the design project, he becomes a member of user group U1 (until he logs off or until his membership in U1 is tested again). If he is using terminal number 42, he also becomes a member of U3 for the present, and so on. If he logs in to use FORTRAN, he will further be a member of U4 and is availed its access rights. The group of all users logging in during the morning is defined by:

$$C(u,U5) : \underline{TIME}(u) < 12{:}\emptyset\emptyset$$

where TIME is the system time-of-day clock and "12:ØØ" denotes noon.

## DATA UNIT DEFINING CONDITIONS

References to data, whether for access or for access control, are very dependent upon the structure of the system environment. A great deal of work by many researchers and designers has been expended on the problem of formulating references to data for storage and retrieval. Their results are equally applicable to the counterpart problem in protection. Taking a relational data base environment as an example, sublanguages--such as SEQUEL [ASTRM74] or SQUARE [BOYCR75]--for expressing queries may also be used to express data definitions for protection. All expressible relations [CODDE7Ø] are valid descriptions of data to be protected. In most real systems it will often be desirable to use a combination of explicit naming and implicit conditional definitions. The explicit naming, such as by providing a file name, describes a domain in which the condition is to be applied.

Here is an example which uses both the file name "personnel" and content values for fields named "dept" and "salary":

$$C(r,R3) = \underline{FILE}(r) = 'personnel' \wedge \underline{dept}(r) = 7 \wedge \underline{salary}(r) < 20000$$
$$\wedge (\underline{FIELD}(r) = 'name' \vee \underline{FIELD}(r) = 'address')$$

Here, the convention of specific user assigned data names being lower case and underlined is followed. In addition, words fixed for a particular system, such as names of types of data units (e.g., FIELD), are in upper case and underlined. Built-in functions (e.g. AVERAGE) will be included in this latter category. The above example of a data defining condition describes the set which is the names and addresses taken from the personnel file of employees in Department 7 having an annual salary of less than $2Ø,ØØØ.

ACCESS CONDITIONS

Access conditions--provisos which must be met before certain accesses are allowed --are likely to be associated with global system variables such as the time-of-day clock, modes of operation, status indicators, flags, and internal codes. Many of these indicators contain information deduced by the data base system about the current transaction. For example, suppose that certain accounting information can be entered only on Fridays. For 1976, this is represented by the following access condition:

$$C(s,S3) : \underline{MOD}\ (\underline{day}(s),\ 7) = 2$$

where MOD is the modulo function and day is the day number on the system calendar (a number from 1 to 365). Since the value of every data element is a direct function of the data base system state, the free variable s can be dropped from the expressions for access conditions. That is, it can be assumed to be attached to every variable in an access condition.

Also, some data content dependent conditions are more appropriate as access conditions than as part of data definitions. For example, if the data base system is capable of synthesizing an average of a certain type of value over a file (as a built-in data base function) in response to a query, the following is an acceptable access condition:

$$\underline{AVERAGE}(\underline{salary}) < 2\text{Ø}\text{Ø}\text{Ø}\text{Ø}$$

The criteria for whether a certain condition is more appropriate as an access condition or as a definition of another set, such as a user group or data unit, are to a large extent implementation questions. As such, the subject is beyond the scope of this paper. Basically, the difference shows up in the time at which the condition is evaluated.

## 3. THE SECURITY SPACE AS A 5-DIMENSIONAL DISCRETE SPACE

### 3.1 DEFINITION OF THE SPACE

If a single element were to be chosen from each of the five basic sets of the model and put together in an ordered 5-tuple:

$$(a,u,e,r,s) \tag{1}$$

where $a\varepsilon\underline{A}$, $u\varepsilon\underline{U}$, $e\varepsilon\underline{E}$, $r\varepsilon\underline{R}$ and $s\varepsilon\underline{S}$, it would represent a single point in a discrete 5-space whose coordinate dimensions correspond to the five sets. The cartesian product of all the sets makes up this entire <u>security space</u>.

ACCESS REQUESTS AND QUERIES

The purpose of a data base system is to serve the user in response to an <u>access request</u> or <u>query</u>. An access request, or query, is a 4-tuple:

$$q = (u,e,R,s)$$

where $u\varepsilon\underline{U}$, $e\varepsilon\underline{E}$, $R\subseteq\underline{R}$, and $s\varepsilon\underline{S}$. This represents a request by an individual user u for a single operation e to a data unit R at a time when the system is in state s. Of the four elements, the user actually provides only the names of e and R. Both u and s are supplied by the system in an "unforgeable" manner.

AUTHORIZATION SPECIFICATIONS

An instance of an authorization specification (or authorization, for short) is a

5-tuple:

$$(a,U,E,R,S) \tag{2}$$

where $a \in \underline{A}$, $U \subseteq \underline{U}$, $E \subseteq \underline{E}$, $R \subseteq \underline{R}$, and $S \subseteq \underline{S}$. This 5-tuple represents a declaration by authorizer a that each and every individual user in group U may do any or all of the operations in E to any or all of the data elements in R only if the system is in one of the states in S.

The basic authorization states who is giving whom the authority to perform what operations on what data units and under what conditions. An authorization permits an authorizer to express the fact that previously established definitions of a user group, a data unit, and an access condition are tied together.

The 5-tuple in (2) is of a different kind than that in (1), because the last four items in (2) are not just elements of their corresponding sets, but are subsets. Therefore, an authorization 5-tuple describes a subspace of the five dimensional security space. Clearly, too, a query is a subspace of a four dimensional projection of the security space. The enforcement problem requires a determination of whether the request is authorized, i.e., whether the access request subspace is completely contained within the subspace characterized by the authorizations.

To help clarify terminology, several similar terms are related here. A protection requirement is a general statement of an authorizer's need. He communicates his need in the syntax of a protection language statement or expression. The syntax of protection language statements may vary widely, but each different form must translate unambiguously into a 5-tuple, which is an authorization specification (or just an authorization).

## EXAMPLE OF AUTHORIZATION SPECIFICATIONS

Consider this protection requirement, taken from [CONWR72]: A user may see and update only "financial" parts of each record in a file, say "personnel," and only between 9 a.m. and 5 p.m. from a specific terminal in the payroll office. Let it also be required that the user be a member of the payroll department. The user group is defined by:

$$C(u,U6) : \underline{\text{dept}}(u)=\text{'payroll'} \wedge \underline{\text{terml}}(u)=\text{'payoffice'}$$

The data unit is:

$$C(r,R5) : \underline{\text{FILE}}(r)=\underline{\text{personnel}} \wedge \underline{\text{FIELD}}(r)=\underline{\text{salary}} \vee \underline{\text{FIELD}}(r)=\underline{\text{rate}})$$

assuming the salary and rate fields are the "financial" part of the records. The access condition is:

$$C(s,S7) : \underline{\text{TIME}} > 9{:}00 \wedge \underline{\text{TIME}} < 17{:}00$$

With these conditions, a subspace of the security space can now be characterized. The subspace corresponds to the authorization which has the following specification:

$$p4 = (a,U6,\{\text{READ},\text{UPDATE}\},R5,S7)$$

## 4. PROCESSES OF THE MODEL

### 4.1 MODELLING THE AUTHORIZATION PROCESS

Before the authorization process translates the protection language expressions of authorizers into internal representations of access control information, it first validates each authorization. The process then handles withdrawing as well as granting of rights, keeps lists of authorizer-created definitions, controls the display of access control information, and keeps a journal of all transactions with the protection system. In this paper, discussion will be limited to the process of validation.

## VALIDATION--THE FIRST STEP

Validation reflects the set of rules governing the various degrees of ownership. There is more than one way to formulate such a set of rules, especially with respect to the role of the SYSADMIN. The following is typical set of validation rules:

1) SYSADMIN is the only authorizer who can assign OWN, and he may do so only if he also owns the data unit specified.

2) An authorizer must own a data unit to grant SUBOWN to it.

3) An authorizer must own or subown a data unit to grant access to it.

A reasonable validation policy must have the general property that ownership (of some kind) of a data unit is a prerequisite for granting authorization to others for its use. Determination of ownership in evaluating validation rules requires invocation of the enforcement process with respect to OWN as a data operation. This will entail the evaluation of an access condition in cases where ownership is conditionally defined.

## 4.2 MODELLING THE ENFORCEMENT PROCESS

The separation of policies and mechanisms in the enforcement process produces some choices to be specified within a given implementation. For example, a result must be defined for the case of two or more authorizations (called <u>matching authorizations</u>) naming the same user group, data operations, and data units. Matching authorizations may have different access conditions. Since it is not useful to interpret such occurrences as conflicts or inconsistencies, they must be treated as modifications of one another. That is, their access conditions must be logically combined, either by an AND or by an OR function. The enforcement process is independent of this choice; rather, it is a matter of policy. If the choice is an OR function, then matching authorizations modify each other by increasing the number of conditions under which access is allowed, forming a less restrictive resultant access condition. If the choice is AND, the matching authorizations modify each other by adding to the conditions which must be satisfied before access is allowed, forming a more restrictive resultant access condition.

Grouping into subsets is also affected by policy. The ability to group users, data elements, and states into possibly non-disjoint subsets of $\underline{U}$, $\underline{R}$, and $\underline{S}$, respectively, is of such importance in real systems that methods for dealing with these groupings must be taken into account. The choice of logical functions to deal with the groupings is a matter of policy. The security space model and its enforcement algorithm are not dependent upon a particular choice, but it is interesting to consider the motivation for and consequences of a given policy. In the next two sections a rationale is given for a particular choice of policy.

## A POLICY FOR OVERLAPPING USER GROUPS--AN OR FUNCTION

The grouping of users is a logical grouping based on common access rights that are not necessarily based on organizational or administrative structure. Since each of the authorization specifications indicates that every member of its group is given certain access rights, an individual in two different groups may gain access via either the access conditions for one group or the access conditions of the other. Thus, an appealing policy choice is to compute the access condition for a single user in two different user groups (with respect to a given data unit and data operation) as the logical OR of the access conditions taken for each group alone.

## A POLICY FOR OVERLAPPING DATA UNITS--AN AND FUNCTION

The definition of an authorization specification (2) imposes necessary conditions for access, but does not constitute sufficient conditions. A later specification naming data elements common to the data units in a previous authorization will have the effect of making more stringent the provisions for access to those common elements. The first specification requires that certain conditions be met and the later specification requires that other conditions must also be met for access to the same data elements. Thus, it might be desirable to compute the new access condition for the common data elements as the logical AND of all the contributing access conditions.

## ADVANTAGES OF THE OR-AND POLICY CHOICE

The choice of logical functions stated above has the following desirable consequences:

1) A single authorization can assign to the GENERAL user group an overall minimum level of rights. The OR function over user groups will merge the GENERAL rights with each user's more specific individual rights.

2) The AND function over data units gives a non-subvertible authority to an owner of a data unit with shared ownership. Each other owner can only make access conditions more restrictive, but can never defeat the intent of an owner by making the conditions less restrictive.

3) In cases where extra precautions are necessary, complete assurance that access to a given data unit is blocked is achieved by a constant "false" access condition in conjunction with the AND function over the resources.

4) A convenient way to refer to <u>exceptions</u> is made possible by the AND function. For example, suppose R2 ⊂ R1 and access is to be granted to all of R1 except R2. This can be done without specifying the elements of R1-R2. Access is authorized in p1 for R1. Then a specification p2, containing a constant "false" access condition, is issued for R2. All requests for R1-R2 will involve only p1 in the access decision. But requests for data elements in R2 will be denied on the basis of the AND of conditions for R1 and the "false" condition for R2.

## THE ENFORCEMENT PROCESS AS A SERIES OF STEPS

Before proceeding with the enforcement process, it is convenient to define some projection functions which operate on n-tuples. In general, where p = (x1,x2,... x[n]), a set of <u>projection functions</u> i(p) = x[i], is defined for i = 1,2,..,n. Since the tuples of this model carry specific element names, mnemonic meaning is better served by the use of the names of the elements instead of a general scheme with subscripts. Therefore, for p = (a1,U3,E7,R4,S6):

a(p) = a1

U(p) = U3

E(p) = E7

R(p) = R4

S(p) = S6

Also, let $\underline{P}$ = {p1,p2,...,p[k]} be the net collection of valid authorization specifications up to a given time. Each element, p, is a 5-tuple of the form (2).

The enforcement process is now stated in the context of a request, q = (u,e,R,s), and the access decision is computed. An example will be developed concurrently to illustrate the application of enforcement.

In the interest of improved readability the algorithm will not include the combining done for matching authorizations. This is a simple function and, in any implementation, would be accomplished by the authorization process before enforcement is activated. Also, the algorithm is simplified by arbitrarily using an OR for the user-group-combining function and an AND for the data-unit-combining function. The reader should note that these are policy choices and a different set of functions could easily be substituted.

Let us assume that, at a given point in time, the following specifications and the associated definitions exist in the system:

$\underline{P}$ = { p1 = (a,U1,e,R2,$\underline{S}$), p2 = (a,U1,e,R3,S1),
p3 = (a,U2,e,R1,S2), p4 = (a,U2,e,R4,S3),
p5 = (a,U3,e,R1,S4), p6 = (a,U4,e,R1,S5),
p7 = (a,U4,e,R2,S6), p8 = (a,U4,e,R3,S7)}

For the purpose of discussion a single authorizer, a, and a single operation, e, are employed. Further, let C[i] be the access condition corresponding to state subset S[i]. The information in $\underline{P}$ can be represented as the matrix of access conditions in Figure 1. Note that this is <u>not</u> what is commonly referred to as an access matrix. (The matrix used here contains access conditions as elements).

| | $R_1$ | $R_2$ | $R_3$ | $R_4$ |
|---|---|---|---|---|
| $U_1$ | 0 | 1 | $C_1$ | 0 |
| $U_2$ | $C_2$ | 0 | 0 | $C_3$ |
| $U_3$ | $C_4$ | 0 | 0 | 0 |
| $U_4$ | $C_5$ | $C_6$ | $C_7$ | 0 |

Figure 1 - Matrix of Access Conditions

Now, consider a request q = (u,e,R,s) such that u(q) ε U2 and u(q) ε U4. Suppose that it is also determined that R(q) has elements in common with R1 and R3.

The enforcement algorithm follows, and each step is in italics to separate it from the related commentary and the application of that step to the example.

(1a) *Determine from the set of known user groups those groups to which the requesting user u(q) belongs.*

(1b) *Collect from P, the set of all authorizations received to date, those authorizations which have the user groups determined in (1a) as elements.*

This set of authorizations is called F(u), the franchise of the user u(q):

$$F(u) = \{p \in \underline{P} : u(q) \in U(p)\}$$

Since, in the example, the requesting user is a member of U2 and U4, F(u) contains all elements of P mentioning U2 or U4:

$$F(u) = \{p3,p4,p6,p7,p8\}$$

(2) *Determine the set of authorizations which have specified e(q) as an elemental operation.*

This set is called the franchise of the operation, F(e):

$$F(e) = \{p \in \underline{P} : e(q) \in E(p)\}$$

In the example e is fixed; therefore F(e) = P.

(3) *Determine the set of authorizations which name data units having elements in common with the requested unit R(q).*

This set is called the franchise of the resource, F(R):

$$F(R) = \{p \in \underline{P} : R(q) \cap R(p) \neq \phi\}$$

Since the requested data are contained in both R1 and R3, F(R) contains all elements of P mentioning R1 or R3:

$$F(R) = \{p2,p3,p5,p6,p8\}$$

(4) *Determine those authorizations common to the three franchises found in steps (1), (2), and (3).*

This set is D(q), the domain of authorization for request q:

$$D(q) = F(u) \cap F(e) \cap F(R)$$

D(q) is the set of all authorizations which relate to the u, e, and R of the request. In this example, the set of all authorizations relating to u (being a member of U2 and U4), to R (overlapping R1 and R2), and to operation e is as follows:

$$D(q) = \{p3,p6,p8\}$$

(5) *Determine the set of all data units named in elements of D(q).*

As this is the data referenced by the query, this set will be called R*, the data reference.

$$R^* = \bigcup_i \{R(p[i]) : p[i] \in D(q)\}$$

For this example,

$$R^* = \{R1,R3\}$$

(6) *Determine if the requested data unit, R(q), is covered by R*; i.e., every element of R(q) must be contained in the data unit of some member of D(q).*

This first level check means that R(q) must be a subset of the union of the elements of the data reference. Otherwise, there cannot be the required access rights and access is immediately denied without further checking. It can be said that the covering check separates the "no's" from the "maybe's".

(7a) *Partition the set D(q) into equivalence classes based on the relation such that two authorizations are in the same class if and only if they specify the same data unit.*

(7b) *Construct a single composite authorization for each equivalence class by performing the logical OR over the access conditions of its elements.*

Each of these classes is for the requesting user u(q). Thus, the new set of authorizations--one per data unit in R*, the data reference--is F(u,q), the <u>effective franchise of the user u(q) with respect to the request q</u>.

Step (7) is accomplished formally as follows:

Let R* = {R1,R2,...,R[r]}. Partition D(q) into r equivalence classes such that the i-th class is:

$$D[i](q) = \{p \in D(q) : R(p)=R[i]\}$$

for i=1,2,...,r. Construct a temporary composite authorization for each class, D[i](q):

$$\hat{p}[i] = (a,u(q),e(q),R[i],\bigcup_j S(p[j] \in D[i](q)))$$

Then $F(u,q) = \{\hat{p}[i] : i=1,2,...,r\}$

Returning to the original example,

$$F(u,q) = \{(a,u(q),e,R1,S2 \cup S5),\ (a,u(q),e,R3,S7)\}$$

The result of this step, as an OR of the user's rights over all groups of which he is a member, is easier to see in the matrix of access conditions, Figure 2.

| | $R_1$ | $R_2$ | $R_3$ | $R_4$ |
|---|---|---|---|---|
| $U_1$ | 0 | 1 | $C_1$ | 0 |
| $U_2$ | $C_2$ | 0 | 0 | $C_3$ |
| $U_3$ | $C_4$ | 0 | 0 | 0 |
| $U_4$ | $C_5$ | $C_6$ | $C_7$ | 0 |

EFFECTIVE FRANCHISE OF u: $C_2 \vee C_5$    $C_7$

Figure 2 - The OR Function Over User Groups

(8) *Find EAC(q), the <u>effective access condition corresponding to the request q</u>, by performing the logical AND over the access conditions of the members of F(u,q).*

The effect is that an AND is taken over all data units which overlap the requested resource unit:

$$EAC(q) = C(s, \bigcap_i S(\hat{p}[i]))$$

For the example,

$$\text{EAC}(q) = C(s, (S2 \cup S5) \cap S7)$$
$$= (C2 \vee C5) \wedge C7$$

The result of this step is shown in Figure 3 as an AND of access conditions over R1 and R3.

| | $R_1$ | $R_2$ | $R_3$ | $R_4$ |
|---|---|---|---|---|
| EFFECTIVE FRANCHISE OF u | $C_2 \vee C_5$ | - | $C_7$ | - |

$$\text{EAC} = (C_2 \vee C_5) \wedge C_7$$

Figure 3 - The AND Function Over Data Units

(9) *Evaluate the effective access condition and render an access decision: permit (the requested access), if EAC holds; deny (the access), if otherwise.*

This step itself might require physical accesses to obtain data contents used in access conditions.

(10) *If the decision is to permit the access, complete the logical access operation by passing the data to or from the user.*

As the above sequence is used mainly for expository reasons, an implementation should not be bound by that sequence. For example, steps (1), (2), and (3) can be done in parallel, or at least progressively such that the results from each step form a starting point (domain) for the next step. In fact, it is expected that much of the procedure can be accomplished in advance, before any requests are considered for enforcement. For example, matching authorizations can be combined, as they enter the system, by the authorization process. The franchise of the user (step (1)) and the effective franchise of the user (step (7)) can be computed as part of the user's log-in procedure and kept for the duration of a session at the terminal.

A relational database system is an ideal environment in which to implement this model. The collection of authorization tuples is a relation. Many of the steps of the enforcement algorithm are nothing more than relational calculus descriptions of queries over this authorization relation, operating on subsets of its tuples.

## 5. ADDITIONAL WORK

Several protection features which may be necessary in a real access control system have not been presented with the basic model, because of space limitations. These features will be reported soon [HARTH76]. A report on the design and application of the protection languages themselves will also be prepared. In addition, work has begun on a study of performance, precision, and cost of protection as a function of the dynamics requirements of enforcement.

Future directions for this research may include a study of protection policies. The model presented here is a general framework of mechanisms in which a large variety of policies can be imbedded. Several studies can benefit from a characterization of the set of possible policies. For example, what is the effect of policy on such factors as the combining of authorizations in the enforcement algorithm and the validation of authorizations in the authorization process?

A further area for study is in the adaption of the model to dynamically adjust authorization information to maintain consistent control over data derived from the database (new files, tables, or views). Some interesting related work has recently been published [DENND76, GRIFP76].

## 6. ACKNOWLEDGEMENTS

The authors wish to thank Professor Douglas S. Kerr, Department of Computer and Information Science, The Ohio State University, for his helpful suggestions during the early stage of this work. Gratitude is also expressed for the excellent suggestions for improvement by the referees.

## REFERENCES

ASTRM74 Astrahan, Morton M., Chamberlin, Donald D., "Implementation of a Structured English Query Language," Comm. ACM 18, 10 (October 1975), 580-588.

BARRD67 Barron, D. W., Fraser, A. G., Hartley, D. F., Landy, B., Needham, R. M., "File Handling at Cambridge University," Proc. SJCC 3Ø (1967), 163-167.

BAUMR75 Baum, R. I., and Hsiao, D. K., "A Semantic Model for Protection Mechanisms in Data Base Systems," Proc. of the Eighth Hawaii International Conference on Systems Sciences (January 1975), 175-179.

BOYCR75 Boyce, R. F., Chamberlin, D. D., Hammer, M. M., and King, W. F. III, "Specifying Queries as Relational Expressions," ACM-SIGPLAN Notices 1Ø. 1 (January 1975)/Sigr Forum IX,3 (Winter 1974), 31 - 47.

BRAND73 Branstad, Dennis K., "Privacy and Protection in Operating Systems," IEEE Workshop, June 12-14, 1972, Princeton, N. J. Reprinted in Computer (January 1973), 43-46.

CODDE7Ø Codd, E., "A Relational Model of Data for Large, Shared Data Banks," Comm. ACM 13, 6 (June 197Ø), 377-387.

CONWR72 Conway, R., Maxwell, W., and Morgan, H., "On the Implementation of Security Measures in Information Systems," Comm. ACM 15, 4 (April 1972), 211-22Ø.

DENND76 Denning, Dorothy E., "A Lattice Model of Secure Information Flow," Comm. ACM 19, 5 (May 1976), 236-242.

DENNJ66 Dennis, J. B., and Van Horn, E. C., "Programming Semantics for Multiprogrammed Computations," Comm. of the ACM 9, 3 (March 1966), 143-155.

DENNJ72 Dennis, Jack B., "On the Design and Specification of a Common Base Language," Project MAC Report MAC TR-1Ø1, M.I.T. (June 1972).

FRIET7Ø Friedman, T. D., "The Authorization Problem in Shared Files," IBM Systems Journal 7, 4 (197Ø), 258-28Ø.

GRAHG72 Graham, G. Scott, and Denning, Peter J., "Protection--Principles and Practice," Proc. SJCC 4Ø (1972), 417-429.

GRIFP76 Griffiths, P. P., and Wade, B. W., "An Authorization Mechanism for a Relational Data Base System," to appear in ACM Transactions on Database Systems.

HANSM71 Hansen, Morris., "Insuring Confidentiality of Individual Records in Data Storage and Retrieval for Statistical Purposes," Proc. FJCC 39 (1971), 579-585.

HARTH75 Hartson, H. Rex, "Languages for Specifying Protection Requirements in Data Base Systems--A Semantic Model," The Ohio State University Computer and Information Science Research Center Report OSU-CISRC-TR-75-6, (August 1975).

HARTH76 Hartson, H. Rex, "Full Protection Specifications in the Semantic Model for Data Base Protection Languages," to appear in Proceedings of the 1976 ACM Annual Conference.

HOFFL69 Hoffman, Lance J., "Computers and Privacy: A Survey," Computing Surveys 1, 2(June 1969), 85-1Ø3 of Computer and Information Science, The Ohio State University (1975).

HSIAD68 Hsiao, D. K., "Access Control in an On-Line System," File Organization--Selected Papers from FILE68--An I.A.G. Conference, Student Literature AB, Lund, Sweden, 1968.

JONEA73 Jones, Anita K., "Protection in Programmed Systems," Ph.D. Dissertation, Department of Computer Science, Carnegie-Mellon University (June 1973).

LAMPB71 Lampson, B. W., "Protection," Proc 5th Princeton Symposium on Information Science and Systems, Princeton University, (March 1971), 437-443. Reprinted in Operating Systems Review 8, 1 (January 1974), 18-24.

SALTJ75 Saltzer, Jerome H., and Schroeder, Michael D., "The Protection of Information in Computer Systems," Proc. of the IEEE, 63, 9 (September 1975), 1278-1308.

WULFW74 Wulf, W., et al "HYDRA: The Kernel of a Multiprocessor Operating System," Comm. ACM 17, 6 (June 1974), 337-344.

*Systems for Large Data Bases, P.C. Lockemann and E.J. Neuhold, (eds.)*
*North-Holland Publishing Company, 1976*

# A TAXONOMY OF DATA MODELS

L.Kerschberg*, A.Klug and D.Tsichritzis
Computers Systems Research Group
University of Toronto
Toronto,Ontario,Canada

This paper classifies a collection of conceptual data models within a taxonomy framework consisting of the following parameters: graph theoretic versus set theoretic models, mathematical foundations, terminology, and semantic levels of abstraction.

## 1. INTRODUCTION

In the last few years there has been a sizable research effort in the area of data models. This is due in part to the importance of the subject conceptually, philosophically and in practice. Before one can attempt to understand, design, implement or simply use a Data Base Management System (DBMS), one needs a data model. In addition, not all people think alike, so that different intellectual tools may appeal to different people. Hence, different data models may be needed.

Many data models have already been proposed, each having its own concepts and terminology. In studying the various models it becomes apparent that they have similarities and differences which are not trivial to analyze. This paper attempts to study a collection of data models using a common framework.

We are not proposing a meta-model capable of capturing all the features of every model. Nor are we promoting any particular model as being the best in any way. Our goal is to point out the concepts and features of each model and how they relate to other models. In this way we hope to aid the prospective data model builder to place his own model in perspective. But most important of all, we hope to help the DBMS user understand what is available so that he may choose his own conceptual tools according to this tastes and needs.

When one considers the many facets of a data model, it soon becomes apparent that a reference frame must be established which is rich enough to differentiate among the various issues involved. In the literature

* Visiting Research Professor. On leave of absence from Computer Science Department, Pontificia Universidade Catolica, Rua Marques de São Vicente, 209, Rio de Janeiro, Brazil. Present Address: Department of Information Systems Management, U. of Maryland, College Park, Md., 20742. This research was sponsored in part by the Canadian National Research Council, FINEP Contract No. 244/CT, IBM of Brazil, Ltd., and IBM of Canada, Ltd.

the data model proponents discuss the relative merits of their models compared to the relative disadvantages of the others. However, one has the feeling that in many cases the comparisons somehow miss the mark, not being able to capture the correct "shades of meaning" or the right "level of abstraction".

Thus, the framework we seek should be able to:

1) Provide the proper "levels of abstraction".
2) Distinguish between seemingly related concepts.
3) Show the equivalence of apparently different concepts.
4) Evaluate all data models objectively.

One important aspect of the classification deals with data model structure. First, we are interested in whether a model has an underlying graph. The graph, while helping to visualize overall information organization, introduces the problem of our understanding the meaning of a node or arc. For example, a node may represent a set, a concept, an event, or a binary relation, while an arc may stand for an attribute, a function, a mapping, a verb, or a structural link. We summarize the graph theoretical terminology in Table I.

Second, the data models without graph structure tend to be set oriented. In these models we are interested in the structure of these sets, ie., whether they are "nested" or "flat".

The mathematical foundations of the data models center on Algebra. Basically, the models can be classified by their use of binary relations, n-ary relations, or a combination of both. A fundamental construct interrelates the various mathematical formulations, namely, that a binary relation from a set A to a set B can be viewed either as a "mapping" of elements of A to those of B, or as a subset (of ordered pairs) of the Cartesian product of A and B.

Next, we study the basic concepts used by the data models, and attempt to establish the similarities and differences among both the concepts and data model terminology.

Lastly, we deal with the semantics of the data models. By "semantics" we mean the extent to which the information structures of a data model convey the meaning of the data contained in the data base.

## 2. THE DATA MODELS UNDER STUDY

In all, we discuss twenty-three data models. We concentrate on the features of fifteen of these. They are:

1. The Relational Data Model (Codd, 1970, 1971)
2. The DBTG/CODASYL Model (CODASYL, 1971)
3. The Hierarchical Model (IMS, System 2000)
4. The DIAM II Model (Senko, 1974)
5. The Infological Model (Langefors, 1974; Sundgren, 1975)
6. The Binary Logical Association Model (Bracchi, et al., 1976)
7. The Entity-Relationship Model (Chen, 1976)
8. Data Semantics (Abrial, 1974)
9. The Functional Data Model (Nijssen, 1975; Kerschberg & Pacheco, 1975)
10. The Semantic Network Model (Roussopoulos & Mylopoulos, 1975)
11. The Extended Set Theory Model (Childs, 1968, 1974)
12. Information Management Concepts (Durchholz and Richter, 1974, 1976)

13. The Information Algebra Model (Kobayashi, 1975, and CODASYL, 1962)
14. The Data Space Model (Bachman, 1973)
15. The Lindgreen Model (Lindgreen, 1974)

An extended version of this paper is available as Tech Report 70 from the Computer Systems Research Group of the U. of Toronto. In it we provide a brief description of each of the above models. Also, we treat logical access mechanisms as another parameter of the framework.

## 3. THE CLASSIFICATION OF THE DATA MODELS

In this section we classify the data models with respect to the taxonomy framework presented earlier. The classification begins with structural comparisons. Here graph theoretic models are compared with set theoretic models. The models are also classified with respect to their use of binary relations, n-ary relations, or a combination of both.

Section 3.2 deals with conceptual comparisons and terminology. Lastly, section 3.3 discusses the "semantics" of data models.

### 3.1. STRUCTURAL COMPARISONS

In this section we isolate and compare the mathematical structure of the data models. Conceptual differences are for the moment ignored. The first analysis sees the models divided into graph theoretic and set theoretic classes. This division is quite natural since some models have an obvious graph structure while those that do not tend to use set operations in a more significant way than the graph models.

First, data models with graph structure are presented. Next we describe the structure of the set theoretic data models. The third sub section presents a partition of the data models based on their use of binary relations, n-ary relations, or a mixture of both. As a result, the evolution of DIAM-I to DIAM-II is easy to understand.

#### 3.1.1. GRAPH THEORETIC MODELS

The nodes of the models are categorized as either structured or unstructured. The structured nodes are types of records or tuples. To represent a structured node in a model with unstructured nodes, new nodes are introduced for each field of the record type and are connected to the original node. The reverse process may be more difficult since it necessitates identifying nodes which are functioning as value sets and ones which are functioning as record types. A process similar to this is described by Adiba et al. (1976). Mathematically, unstructured nodes are just point sets.

The edges represent the means for moving from node to node. We are viewing the nodes as sets and we can view the edges also as mathematical objects, namely binary relations. As such it is meaningful to consider the functionality of the edges.

Four of the models have functional edges: the DBTG model, the Hierarchical Model, the Functional Model and the Entity-Relationship Model. In the traditional way of drawing DBTG and Hierarchical diagrams, the edge points from the range to the domain of the function. The Functional Model has the edges pointing from domain to range, the usual custom in mathematics. The functions of the Hierarchical and Functional Models are total while those of the DBTG Model may be partial. Nijssen (1975)discusses how DBTG owner coupled sets may be viewed as functions.

Non-functional edges are also represented by directed edges. Mathematically, the relation may not be symmetric. Hence the roles of the two nodes are different and this is indicated by an asymmetric, i.e., directed, edge. Some models have a different graphic notation but the effect is the same. If the relation happens to be functional, the arrow usually points in the functional direction.

Graphs of models having only functional edges may also be represented in a graph model with non-functional edges without changing the graph structure. This disregards differences in node structure. The converse problem, that of representing non-functional edges in a graph having only functional edges, is a bit more difficult. For a non-functional edge, a new node is created (the link record type) which mathematically is the set of ordered pairs characterizing the non-functional edge. The new node is connected to the original nodes by new functional edges which mathematically are projections.

The graphs of the Entity-Relationship Model are tripartite, that is, there are three classes of nodes and edges only connect nodes of different classes. If we ignore the value nodes, a relationship set corresponds to a DBTG "link record" type (Durchholz, 1975). Chen's relationship sets, however, have severe restrictions on their allowed connections to other nodes (sets), while DBTG link record types may be connected freely to other nodes.

There are two models which place restrictions on edge occurrences: the Hierarchical and Entity-Relationship Models. The graph of the Hierarchical Model must be a collection of trees, while in the latter model's graph, participant edges connect only relationship sets with entity sets. Attribute edges of these sets are incident to value sets.

Also, Steel (1975) has recommended that the restriction that D B T G cosets connect different record types be removed, since it is mainly an implementation restriction. The models described by directed graphs or sets are classified in Tables 1 and 2, respectively.

### 3.1.2. SET THEORETIC MODELS

Although the tuple also embodies data relationships in graph models with structured nodes, in set theoretic models the tuple is the principle vehicle for representing relationships. We use two parameters for subdividing the set models. We group them according to tuple size and according to set nesting. Each model either has a nested or a flat structure.

By nested structure we mean that elements of tuples can themselves be sets. The three models with nested structure are the Information Management Concepts, Extended Set Theory and the Hierarchical Relational Model. The first two are very similar in their structure. Collections correspond to sets and nominations correspond to tuples. The elements of a nomination are selected by names while the elements of a tuple are selected by natural numbers. The main difference between selection by name and selection by natural number is that any tuples of the same size have the same selectors, while two nominations can have none, some or all of their selectors the same. The complexes of Extended Set Theory do not have a counterpart in the Durchholz and Richter Model.

Table 1: GRAPH THEORETIC MODELS

| | MODEL | NODE | NODE ELEMENT | EDGE | FUNCTIONALITY |
|---|---|---|---|---|---|
| structured node elements | DBTG | Record Type | Record | (Co) Set Type | member → owner (against arrow) |
| | Hierarchical | Segment Type | Segment | Parent/Child Relationship | child → parent (against arrow) |
| | General Network | Record Type | Record | Link | none |
| | Information Algebra (Kobayashi) | Area | Point | Arc | none |
| unstructured node elements | DIAM-II | Identifier | Id. Value | Association Pair | none |
| | Binary Logical Associations | Set of Concepts | Concept | Logical Association | none |
| | Abrial's | Category | Object | Relation | none |
| | Functional | Set | Entity,<br>Abstract Entity,Value | Function | domain → range (with arrow) |
| multiple node types | Entity-Relationship | Value Set<br>Entity Set<br>Relationship Set | Value<br>Entity<br>Relationship | Attribute<br>Role | Attr: ES → VS<br>Attr: RS → VS<br>Role: RS → ES |
| | Semantic Network | Value Node<br>Concept Node<br>Event Node<br>Characteristic Node | Value<br>"Entity"<br>Event<br>Property | Characteristic<br>Role<br>Characteristic | ch: Char. node → Concept<br>ch: Char. node → Event<br>v: Char. node → Value |

When we say that a model has a flat structure we mean that the elements of tuples are "simple" objects. Unnormalized relations and the e-messages of the Infological Model are, precisely speaking, not flat. However, it is not proper to call them nested structures. Rather, they are the result of bracketed Cartesian products, which Codd (1971a) refers to as "factorization".

The flat models are further divided according to the size of the tuples they use. We will first discuss the models with tuples of arbitrary length.

The Relational, Information Algebra and Infological models all use arbitrarily sized tuples. It is convenient to consider the Relational Model as middle ground and to relate the other two models to it.

The e-concept of the Infological Model is approximately equivalent to a relation. The e-concept defines an e-message type and all e-messages of this type can be considered tuples of the corresponding relation. However, the e-messages still contain the relation or property name as part of their structure. This difference is not really significant, though, because Infological e-messages and tuples of a relation are not at the same level of abstraction. At the Datalogical level, e-messages are represented by e-records which do not contain the relation or property name and therefore are equivalent to tuples.

The time dimension of e-messages is significant. The relations in a relational data base are time-varying and they represent the current state of the world. The e-messages in an Infological data base are also time-varying. However, an e-message can represent a past, present or future fact and its presence in the data base signifies that the fact is known.

In the Information Algebra Model there is only one set of tuples, the information space. Since there is a coordinate in the space for every attribute of every entity represented, null values are provided when the attribute is not applicable. The information space can be thought of as a conglomeration of a number of relations. Each tuple has been extended by null values to include all of the attributes of the other relations. The areas of the information space corresponding to relations can be identified by an appropriate function of areas.

The three models we discuss next all use triplets as the basic information unit.

The Data Space Model and Lindgreen's Model are very similar. The components of the triplets have the names <entity, attribute, measure and <entity, property, value>, respectively. The geometric view of the Data Space Model is contrasted against the more set-theoretic view of Lindgreen's Model. The iso-entity plane and the iso-attribute plane of the Data Space Model are equivalent, respectively, to the isonymous information set and the isotypic information set of Lindgreen's Model. In the Data Space Model the concept of measure is at full parity with the concepts of entity and attribute. Thus the model also uses iso-measure planes to which there is no equivalent in Lindgreen's Model.

DIAM-II is the successor of the original DIAM-I as reported by Senko et al. (1973). It is interesting to note the correspondence in the structure of the two models.

When DIAM-I was being developed, it was considered whether the binary

Table 2: SET THEORETIC MODELS

| MODEL | TUPLE SIZE | NESTING |
|---|---|---|
| Relational | arbitrary | flat |
| Infological | arbitrary | flat |
| Information Algebra | arbitrary | flat |
| I M C | arbitrary | nested |
| Extended Set Theory | arbitrary | nested |
| Hierarchical Relations | arbitrary | nested |
| DIAM-I | triplet | flat |
| Data Space | triplet | flat |
| Lindgreen's | triplet | flat |

association was the most desirable form for the description of entities. Although it was recognized then that a fact is descriptive of both entities (n-ary facts will be discussed below), binary associations were considered to necessitate the introduction of too many names into the system. An asymmetrical representation of facts was chosen, namely the entity description. Very briefly, an entity is described by an entity description which consists of a set of name triplets representing elementary properties or facts. Each triplet contains a Name Set Name, a Role Name, and an Entity Name taken from the Name Set. Descriptions of entities from the same entity set are gathered into a description set with a system-unique name.

The binary form for associations was choosen for DIAM-II to remove two representation dependent aspects of DIAM-I. First, in DIAM-I, a query must specify a description set name rather than the name of the entity set (identifier name) for which the query requests information. Second, the sometimes arbitrary decision of which of the two possible places to store a fact must be made.

DIAM-II resolves these difficulties by removing descriptions and description sets. The name triplet has become the association pair. Role names in DIAM-I correspond to association names in DIAM-II. The naming problem is minimized by realizing that association names need be unique only within the set of association names emanating from a particular identifier. Associations in DIAM-II always come in pairs, i.e., facts have a symmetric representation in DIAM-II and so there is no question about where a fact should be stored. Making triplets symmetric removes the distinction between an entity and a value, as both are treated as entities.

The structure of DIAM-I can also be correlated with that of Lindgreen's Model. By rewriting the DIAM-I Name_Set_Name/Role_Name/Entity_Name triplets in the form Role_Name/(Name_Set_Name)/Entity_Name, we may note the correspondence between a DIAM-I entity description and an isonymous information set from which the entity has been factored. The Role Name corresponds to a property and the Entity Name corresponds to a value. The Name Set Name may also be considered part of the value, but it more closely matches the formal value set of the property. The described entity appears explicitly in a factored isonymous information set. The entity to which a description refers is specified by one (or more) of the triples acting as identifiers. The information as to which of the triples identify the entity must be kept in a Description Set Catalog. Entity descriptions for entities from the same entity set are collected into Description Sets which correspond to homogeneous information sets.

The three models presented here which use triples as the basic information unit can be ordered according to their treatment of the three coordinates. The Data Space Model is the most homogeneous. The entity, attribute and measure coordinates are treated on an equal basis. In Lindgreen's Model entity and property are dealt with similarly. For instance, a homogeneous information set may be factored as a collection of isonymous information sets or as a collection of isotypic information sets. In DIAM-I entities have precedence. There is no primitive notion corresponding to an isotypic information set.

### 3.1.3. MATHEMATICAL STRUCTURE

Instead of classifying models as to their graph theoretic or set theoretic structure, we can study the way they relate "things" in the model. By things we mean entities, data items, values, etc. A data model can relate things in three possible ways: binary relations, n-ary relations, or a combination of both. The grouping of models according to this scheme is presented in Table 3.

Table 3: MATHEMATICAL STRUCTURE-BINARY AND/OR N-ARY

| BINARY | N-ARY | BINARY + N-ARY |
|---|---|---|
| Data Space | Relational | DBTG |
| Lindgreen's | Information Algebra (CODASYL) | Information Algebra (Kobayashi) |
| DIAM-I | Infological | General Network |
| DIAM-II | | Semantic Network |
| Binary Logical Association | | Hierarchical |
| Abrial's | | Hierarchical Relations |
| Functional | | Information Management Concepts |
| | | Extended Set Theory |

In Binary models, things are related in pairs only. The triplet set models and the graph models with unstructured nodes are brought together in the binary relation group. The close relationship of these two classes is emphasized by the presence of both DIAM-I and DIAM-II. The main distinction between the Graph Theoretic and the Set Theoretic subclasses of the Binary group is that the set models maintain asymmetric concepts of "thing being described" and "thing describing", while the graph models treat the two connected things as being equally important. These views will be compared when we make conceptual comparisons.

Another characteristic of the Binary models is the presence or absence of functionalities. The homogeneous information sets of Lindgreen have only one value associated with each property of the entities in the entity spectrum of the HIS. Thus a property can be considered a function from the entity spectrum of the HIS to the value set of the property. In an entity description of DIAM-I a Role Name appears only once. Hence, a Role Name defines a function with a description set as domain and a Name Set as range. The third model with functionalities is, of course, the Functional Model.

The other four models do not use functional relations. The Data Space Model allows multivalued attributes, and DIAM-II, the BLA Model and Abrial's Model permit many-to-many associations.

The models catagorized as N-ary are the Relational Model, CODASYL's Information Algebra and the Infological Model. Things are related in these models by various forms of the tuple. In the Information Algebra and Relational Models it is data items which are related by tuples. The Infological Model relates objects by tuples. Property-type e-messages in this model have similarities with binary relations. However, the attribute-value structure of properties is de-emphasized and property-type e-messages can be considered unary relations.

Data models in the third category relate things in both a binary and an N-ary fashion. As occurred with the Binary group, subclasses of graph theoretic and set theoretic models are grouped together.

At the top of the Binary N-ary classification list we find the General Network (Tsichritzis, 1975), Semantic Network, DBTG, and the Information Algebra models. The n-ary relationships are represented by event nodes, record types, and areas. The binary relationships are the roles, links, and structures. Between any two record types (areas) any number of links (structures) may be defined.

At the bottom of this list are the IMC and Extended Set Theory models. The single binary relationship is set membership. Set membership defines the existence of the enclosing set or construct, as the enclosing set's very identity depends on its members. There can be at most one membership relation between any two sets or constructs.

In the middle of the list are the Hierarchical and Hierarchical Relational models. These models have certain qualities mentioned for the other subcategories. Namely, they are similar to Extended Set Theory and Information Management Concepts (IMC) in that there can be at most one binary relationship between two segment types or relations. On the other hand, the existence of the superior segment (relation) is not predicated upon the existence of its subordinate segments (relations).

It may be argued that sets also represent relationships in models of the other categories. However, sets in these models serve more as cataloging devices, factoring out information commom to the elements of the set. For example, all the sets constituting relations in a relational data base can be mapped onto a single information space of Information Algebra. The identity of the relations is preserved by a function of areas.

## 3.2. CONCEPTUAL COMPARISONS

In section 3.1 we made comparisons based on the mathematical structure of the models. In that section conceptual differences in the things we compared were ignored. For example, the e-messages of the Infological Model were compared with the tuples of the Relational Model. In this section we take note of the concepts which overlay the mathematical structures of the models. Since a model's conceptual organization effects its mathematical structure, there will be some overlap with the discussion of section 3.1.3. However, here the emphasis will be on concepts, their meaning and their implications.

For most of the models the real world is given structure with the concepts of entity, property, value and relationship. The variations of these concepts among the models are two-fold. First there are differences in terminology. Comparable terms are listed in Table 4. The second, more substantial differences involve concept usage. Some models do not employ all concepts and the ones that are used are not used equivalently.

The first question we should ask is, what is an entity? Dictionary definitions are generally used as a first approximation. An entity is something that has reality and distinctness of being in fact or in thought. Of course, the same can be said for properties, values and relationships. What distinguishes entities from the others is not something intrinsic but something subjective: interest. An entity has interest for the individual or enterprise. Relationships, properties and values are also of interest, but only to the degree they provide information about entities.

Some models use entities and relationships only. DIAM and Abrial's model are among these. The requirement that entities be of interest has taken less importance in these models since there is no separate class of values. This is justified in DIAM-I by noting that something like "red" might be of interest, even if it isn't at the moment. Abrial does distinguish between concrete and abstract objects. Abstract objects correspond roughly to values, but concrete objects are definitely entities.

In some sense the Relational Model also is in this category. Specifically, the Relational Model can be said to talk about only values and relationships. This is so because relations represent the *intension* as well as the *extension* of the data, i.e., the meaning and representation of the data.

The next group of models has entities, properties and values. It includes the Data Space Model, CODASYL's Information Algebra and Lindgreen's Model. Since entities can be related only through their properties, the concept of identifier is necessary at the conceptual level. An identifier is any property which puts the value set in one-to-one correspondence with the entities having the property.

The Infological Model and Kobayashi's Information Algebra are examples of models in which entities have properties and may also participate in relations.

Among those models using entities, properties, values and relationships, Chen's Entity-Relationship Model is the most general. Here both entities and relationships have properties.

The concept of entity set or entity type is important in many models. This concept is related to that of property, and the relationship takes one of two forms. Either entity sets are first distinguished and then a set of applicable properties is defined, or else the totality of properties is defined and the entity sets are defined as common domains of certain groups of properties. By defining properties first, the notion of a collection of entity sets having common properties is quite natural. On the other hand, by defining the entity sets first, the sets are not dependent on their properties and consequently properties may easily be added or removed.

If a model has the notion of entity type, the notion a subtype of an entity must be considered. The possibility of overlapping entity types can also arise. Moulin et al. (1976) require that entity sets be disjoint. Their reasons are that this allows unambiguous naming of entities and that relationships cannot be masked by an entity set. It has been noted (Brown, 1975), however, that disjoint entity types can cause too many types to be declared for effective control. DIAM-I notes that one entity type is often a subset of another entity type. For example, a manager is also an employee and has properties ordinary employees do not. The more general case is that of two overlapping entity sets, neither contained in the other. For instance, in a motion picture company, the set of actors and the set of directors overlap. Hall et al. (1976) have noted that the collection of entity sets should be closed under the usual set operations of union, intersection and difference. Chen also notes that entity sets need not be disjoint. None of these models, however, effectively deals with the naming problem referred to by Moulin. No provision is made at representation level for indicating that an entity belongs to two or more entity sets. An entity is generally represented by, or at least identified by, exactly one value from one of a disjoint set of domains.

The basic definition of entities as the main objects of interest with properties, values and relationships subordinate to them is modified when relationships are allowed to have properties as in the models of Chen, Hall et al., and Benci et al. (1976). Without relationship properties, when a relationship becomes interesting in itself it becomes an entity and the roles played by each entity in the relationship now themselves become relationships. Such changes in the model may be avoided by letting relationships become interesting with their own properties without requiring that they become entities.

There are now just two differences between entities and relationships. Relationships can only exist when the related entities also exist and relationships cannot themselves partake in relationships. The first difference is inherent in the meaning of relationship. The second difference is actually a restriction of the particular models. In fact, the Infological model and any model admitting unnormalized relations will allow relationships among relationships. As expected, having relationships with or without properties, among or not among other relationships does not affect the expressive power of the model but it does affect the presence of so-called excess entities (Hall et al. 1976).

Some models allow qualifications in the dependence of relationships on the existence of the participating entities. Sometimes a role in a relationship may be allowed to be vacant. For example, relational attributes not participating in the prime key may have null values. In the other direction, a role may be allowed to have more than one participating entity. For instance, Abrial uses the example: "Peter was invited by Paul and Jane to Paris on July the 15th of 1973."

Excess entities are entities in which there is no real interest but which must be defined because of some restriction in the model. A related notion is that of an excess relationship, that is, a relationship connecting two entities, one of which was formerly a relationship. We stress that the concepts of excess entity and excess relationship are subjective ideas. Moreover, they do have important semantic interpretations, as will be seen shortly.

The only entity model which does not need excess entities is the Infological Model. All e-messages are important to the Infological model, so that excess entities do not arise.

Brown (1975) has described a real world model intended to be mapped to the DBTG model. In models such as this, excess entities occur when nonfunctional relationships must be expressed as entities with domains connected to the relationship entities by what are essentially projections. The Entity-Relationship and Functional Models also use this construct.

Another kind of excess entity occurs when the model only has binary relationships. In this case an n-ary relationship must appear as an entity. The role of each entity in this relationship is now itself a relationship.

With these two kinds of excess entity the term "excess" is in some sense objective because it may very well be that no one is interested in the entities created. It may also happen that one application becomes interested in a relationship and gives it a property or involves it in a relationship. If the model requires that the relationship become an entity there may be other applications which consider this an excess entity. Senko (1975b) has defined a VIA option in the FORAL language which allows excess entities to be skipped over. Thus applications not interested in an entity need not see it.

It is often said that, because a binary relationship is many-to-many, it can become an entity in its own right with its own properties. This is misleading. By the process of abstraction, any (binary) relationship can become an entity. However, if a functional binary relationship has properties of interest, but one does not desire that it become an entity, its properties may be attributed to the entities in its domain without losing any information. Two problems can arise when one attributes properties of a function to its domain. First, if the function is not total, the property is forced to assume null values. Second, if the function is one-to-one, the arbitrary decision must be made whether the property will be attributed to the domain, the range or both. This, of course, is not possible with many-to-many relationships.

We have noted that relationships can have qualities very much like entities, and that they differ mainly in their dependence on the existence of the related entities. It is also possible for entities to have such existence dependence. This dependence may be genuine as in the case of an n-ary relationship entity in a binary model or the dependence may really mean that the interest of one entity depends on the interest in others. Chen defines such dependent entities. For example, an employee's children are only of interest while the employee works for the company. This qualified interest is similar to the interest in values describing entities. Thus dependent entities resemble in some respects values. Deheneffe et al. (1974) also define existence properties of entities.

Schmid and Swenson (1975) have defined a real world view for representation by relations which is based on existence dependence of objects. In this view the world consists of 1) independent objects have an existence of their own and which may enter into associations with one another and, 2) characteristic objects which exist only while they are the describing parts of characteristic relationships. Characteristic objects can have characteristics but cannot be associated with other objects. There are two ways to describe this model in the entity-property-relationship terminology. We can say that the independent objects are the entities and the characteristic objects are the properties. Then we have a model in which properties themselves have properties. Alternatively, both independent and characteristic objects can be two classes of entities; associations and characteristic relationships are two types of relationships and there are no properties. Then we have one class of entity with existence dependencies. We chose the first alternative in listing this model in Table 4. Note that the Semantic Network Model also allows characteristics of characteristics.

The question of when entities are recognized to exist is related to the ability to identify or name them. We distinguish three ways to relate existence and identifiers. The most restrictive is to specify that every entity set must have a set of identifying properties. For example, in DIAM-I every entity description must contain at least one identifier. If all the properties of an entity type are included in the set of identifying properties, we are regarding an entity as the bundle of property values associated with it (Langefors, 1966). Information Algebra is an example of this approach.

A less restrictive way is to allow an entity to be identified by its properties and relationships with other entities. As we have already noted, Chen's dependent entities are of this type. The identity, and therefore the existence, of this type of entity is then dependent on other entities.

A number of models recognize the existence of entities which are not determined uniquely by their properties or relationships. This does not cause any difficulties at the conceptual level. For example, it is easy to visualize a bin full of identical shirts. Special considerations must be taken, however, when representing possibly nondistinguishable entities. To represent such entities, Hall et al. use the notion of surrogate. Abrial's model has internal names. Benci et al. use the concept of entity, but with a connotation different from the one we have used thusfar. These internal identifiers are values, each of which represents one entity, but which have no meaningful external form. One unanswered question concerning nondistinguishable entities is how their representations are manipulated inside the data base. If it is planned that certain entities be nondistinguishable, the concept of a group entity might be needed. Benci's notion of "measure of existence" is somewhat similar. If nondistinguishable entities appear at random, for example, multiple voters registering with the same name and address, there is no way to handle them separately without adding an artificial distinguishing property.

The discussion so far in this section has considered various aspects of the entity concept as they appear in different models. The entity concept, however, is not universally accepted as an appropriate paradigm.

Bracchi et al. (1976) explicitly reject the idea of entity at the conceptual schema level. Their model is based on binary relations defined over "Sets of Concepts". The exact nature of a "Concept" is not specified but one characteristic is that it is the smallest unit of information which is amenable to processing. The proper place for entities is in application views. Concepts serve as basic building blocks for entities. The authors do allow concepts in the conceptual schema model to be built up from more elementary concepts. For example, a DATE is built up from a DAY, a MONTH and a YEAR.

Durchholz and Richter never even use the term "entity". Information is structured directly by the concept of "construct". Projecting structure onto the real world is not necessary in this model because the model is intended to be a conceptual system to describe the universe of discourse between the users and the DBMS. If the user wants to communicate in terms of entities, this structure is built on top of the construct structure.

The extended Set Theory Model of Childs goes even further and views every level of abstraction in terms of sets. Any conceptual structure the user wishes may be built on top of this. Thus constructs, sets of concepts or entities could be defined set theoretically.

T. B. Steel (1975) has also rejected the notion of entity as part of a formalism for the conceptual level. His view is that set theory

Table 4: CONCEPTUAL EQUIVALENTS & TERMINOLOGY

| MODEL | ENTITY | RELATIONSHIP | TYPE* | PROPERTY/APPLICABLE TO |
|---|---|---|---|---|
| Abrial-Data Semantics | Object | Relation | b | ——— |
| DIAM I & II | Entity | Association | b | ——— |
| Lindgreen's | Entity | ——— | ——— | Property/Entity |
| Data Space | Entity | ——— | ——— | Attribute/Entity |
| Information Algebra (CODASYL) | Entity | ——— | ——— | Property/Entity |
| Information Algebra (Kobayashi) | Entity | Arc | b | Property/Entity |
| Benci et al. | Object | Association | n | Property/Object, Association |
| Entity-Relationship | Entity | Relationship | n | Attribute/ Entity, Relationship |
| Infological | Object | Relation | n | Property/Object |
| Schmid & Swenson | Indep. Object | Association | n | Characteristic/Indep. or Char. Object |
| Semantic Network | Concept | Event | n | Characteristic/Concept,Event, Characteristic. |
| Functional | Entity | Abstract Entity | n | Function/Entity or Ab. Entity |

* b denotes a binary relationship
n denotes an n-ary relationship

embedded in a modal logic is the proper choice. The argument, like that of Child's, is that only set theory is sufficiently general to satisfy all modelling requirements.

## 3.3. THE SEMANTICS OF DATA MODELS

Data model proponents all claim that their models capture the "semantics" of data, and for the most part, they do precisely that. By the semantics of data we mean the "meaning" of the data. But just what is the meaning of data? What form does it take? Perhaps an analogy might help in clarifying this point.

The Renaissance sculptor Michealangelo is attributed to have said that when he viewed large blocks of Carrara marble, he could "see" the figures contained within. His role was to "liberate" these forms.

In our analogy a large block of marble corresponds to unstructured data items (raw data) and the finished "liberated" sculpture to the information structures which give meaning or form to the data.

Although this analogy does provide some insight into information structure, it insufficient to be used as a basis for comparison among the data models. A more fruitful approach may be found in linguistics.

One linguistic approach to semantics is Predication Analysis (Leech, 1974). Predication Analysis deals with the semantic structure of sentences. The analysis process involves the identification of the arguments and predicates of a predication. A predication has one predicate and may have zero, one, or two arguments. Moreover, the arguments may themselves be predications, thereby allowing tree structures to be built up. Further, certain predications, called downgraded predications, are the semantic equivalents of the adjective and adverbial functions of syntax. Those predications representing the adjective functions of syntax qualify arguments while those representing the adverbial functions of syntax modify predicates. For example, the sentence

"Suppliers supply parts to departments in specific volume",

would be analyzed as follows:

1. The main predication structure is "suppliers supply parts" with suppliers and parts serving as arguments and the verb supply being the predicate of the predication.

2. The prepositional phrases "to departments" and "in specific volume" are downgraded predications performing the adverbial functions of syntax. Moreover, these downgraded predications modify the predicate "supply".

If we study how the models represent the main predication and its associated downgraded predications, we should be able to conclude how they map the semantic predication structures into information structures. It results that, depending on the model, these information structures embody various semantic "levels of abstraction" which range from surface semantics to deep semantics.

Thus we can introduce the notion of a semantic spectrum, and ask where a data model fits along this spectrum. Those models which use an underlying graph to denote overall information structure are easy to compare, although the graph structure is not essential in capturing data semantics. However, the existence of a graph requires that we know the meaning attached to a node or an arc. In this section we are concerned with how these nodes and arcs model the semantics of the original sentence.

Those models which most closely resemble the surface semantics of a sentence (or a complete discourse) are the Entity-Relationship model and the Semantic Network model. Our example sentence would be modelled by Chen as a ternary relationship involving supplier, part and department entities. The relationship set would be named SUPPLIER-PART-DEPARTMENT and would be connected via undirected arcs to the corresponding entity sets. The downgraded predication representing the volume supplied would be abstracted to an attribute, VOLUME, of the relationship.

The Semantic Network model would view the first predication as the event node SUPPLY connected to the concept nodes supplier, part and departments by arcs labelled agent, object and destination, respectively. The volume supplied is a characteristic of the event node.

Both models consistently identify relationship sets or event nodes with verbs. At times this seems a bit artificial, especially when the relationship is functional, eg., "Every employee is managed by a unique employee". The Entity-Relationship Model creates a relationship set named MANAGEMENT connected to the EMPLOYEE entity set by two arcs labelled MANAGED and MANAGER. Chen argues that although a relationship may be functional at present, i.e. N:1, it may become relational, i.e., N:M, and should therefore be modelled as a relationship. A more convincing argument might be that he is trying to model semantic surface structure.

Another class of models captures some aspects of both surface and deep semantic structure. By deep structure we mean that functional predications such as MANAGEMENT are represented by arcs (properties, attributes, functions) rather than nodes (relations, relationships, sets). Thus in graph models, arc labels may be verb phrases since the node representing the verb may be eliminated. The models in this class are the DBTG/CODASYL, Relational, Infological, and Functional.

The relations of the Relational and Infological models represent semantic "fragments" corresponding to arguments and predications. The attributes of predication relations represent adverbial information as well as "logical pointers" to argument relations. In the DBTG and Functional models, the arcs between predication nodes and argument nodes provide the same semantic structural information given by the "logical pointers" of the non-graph models.

Note however that it is possible to convert the models of this mixed class to strict surface semantics by including relations or nodes representing these functional predications. Mathematically, this corresponds to viewing a binary relation as a set of ordered pairs rather than as a mapping.

At the deep semantic level we have the DIAM-II, Data Semantics, and Binary Logical Association models. At this level the data items or values are viewed as entity sets or Sets of Concepts related by means of binary relations. In these models predication nodes are unnecessary as long as the predications have no downgraded predications (adverbial information) modifying them. In this case they are binary relations, but when adverbial information such as "to departments" and "volume" must be represented, these models create an "excess" node and relate adverbial information to that node. In Senko's FORAL language, a VIA option is provided to skip over these "excess" entities because his language does not use verbs. However, from the semantic point of view these "excess" nodes are important since they are the natural place to attach downgraded predications.

Models such as Information Management Concepts, Information Algebra, and Extended Set Theory actually span all semantic levels of abstraction due to their purely set theoretic nature. Thus these models can be used to construct the view which best suits a particular application. We term these semantics "Preverbal" since non-verbal thought processes are involved in obtaining these data model information structures.

To summarize, we note that surface semantic models capture the way we speak and communicate verbally with one another. The mixed semantic level represents functional relationships as properties of an entity. Lastly at the deep semantic level, entities relinguish their importance to data items which are treated as entities. Associations among entities (in graph models) are labelled with long verb phrases which describe the relationship.

Although the notion of a semantic spectrum is strictly a conceptual device, it does help to explain variations among models which cannot easily be expressed in terms of structural or conceptual comparisons.

Table 5: DATA MODEL SEMANTIC STRUCTURE

| SEMANTIC LEVEL | MODEL |
| --- | --- |
| Surface Semantic | Entity-Relationship<br>Semantic Network<br>Benci et al. |
| Mixed Semantic | Infological<br>Relational<br>DBTG/CODASYL<br>Functional |
| Deep Semantic | Data Semantics<br>DIAM-II<br>Hierarchical<br>Binary Logical Associations |
| Pre-verbal Semantic* | Extended Set Theory<br>Information Management Concepts<br>Data Space<br>Lindgreen's<br>Information Algebra |

* Refers to thought processes other than verbal ones.

## 4. CONCLUSIONS

In this paper we have presented a taxonomy framework for the classification of a collection of conceptual data models. The framework parameters are: structural properties, conceptual comparisons and terminology, and the semantics of data models.

In studying the structural properties of data models, one immediately notices that some provide an underlying graph, while others do not. For models which have a graph we indicate the meanings associated with the nodes and arcs in Table 1. Models not using a graph representation tend to be more set theoretic. They differ in the way the sets are organized as to tuple size and whether these tuples are flat or nested. A classification of these models is given in Table 2.

Another structural aspect of a data model is its mathematical structure. We have found that the models use either binary relations, n-ary relations, or a combination of both. Table 3 provides a classification of the models as to mathematical structure.

One of the most difficult parameters of our taxonomy framework is that of conceptual comparisons and terminology. This parameter is so difficult to handle because 1) models use different terminology to describe the same concept, and 2) the same terminology is sometimes used to describe different concepts. One of the basic findings of our examination of terminology is that some models introduce the notion of an entity while others do not. For those that do use this notion, we found that various forms of the triplet "entity-relationship-property" were common to them. Table 4 provides a listing of those models using entities and the terminology they use in describing the "entity-relationship-property" triplet.

The last component of our framework deals with the semantics of the data models. The models can be classified initially into two classes: those which follow a "subject-predicate-object" semantic approach, and those that do not. To those models falling into the first category, we further refine the classification based on whether the models capture either surface semantics, deep semantics, or a mixture of both. Further, some models use pre-verbal semantics in formulating information structures. Table 5 places the data models along this "semantic spectrum".

We feel that this paper offers several original contributions. To our knowledge, this is the first attempt to classify such a large collection of data models. Moreover, the taxonomy framework helps to clarify the structural aspects of data models and their implications to logical access. By comparing terminology among models, we further refine the conceptual similarities and differences. Lastly, the semantics of data models has been formalized using semantic predication analysis and the notions of surface and deep semantics. The transformation from surface to deep semantics parallels the mathematical approach to viewing a binary relation as a set (of ordered pairs) or as a mapping, respectively.

As stated in the introduction, we do not propose a meta-data model, nor do we suggest that any one model is better than the others. However, we have attempted to provide a framework in which the reader can meaningfully evaluate the data models, and perhaps classify his own.

REFERENCES

Abrial, J.R. (1974) "Data Semantics", Data Base Management, J.W. Klimbie and K.L. Koffeman (eds.), North Holland, 1974.

Adiba, M., Delobel, C. and Leonard, M. (1976) "A unified approach for modelling data in logical data base design", Proc. IFIP-TC-2-WC, Black Forest.

Bachman, C.W. (1973) "Data space mapped into three dimensions", Infotech State of the Art Report 15.

Benci, E., Bodart, F., Bogaert, H. and Cabanes, A. (1976) "Concepts for the design of a conceptual schema", Proc. IFIP-TC-2-WC, Black Forest.

Bracchi, G., Fedeli, A., and Paolini, P. (1972) "A language for a relational data base management system", Princeton Conf. on Information Sciences and Systems 1972.

Bracchi, G., Paolini, P. and Pelagatti, G. (1976) "Binary logical associations in data modelling", Proc. IFIP-TC-2-WC, Black Forest.

Brown, A.P.G. (1975) "Modelling a real world system and designing a schema to represent it", Data Base Description, Douque and Nijssen (eds.), North Holland, 1975.

Boyce, R.F. et al. (1975) "Specifying queries as relational expressions", CACM, 18, 621-628.

Chamberlin, D. and Boyce, R. (1974) "SEQUEL: A structured english query language", ACM SIGMOD-74.

Chen, P. (1976) "The entity-relationship model: toward a unified view of data", to appear TODS 1, # 1.

Childs, D.L. (1968a) "Feasibility of a set-theoretic data structure - - a general structure based on a reconstituted definition of relation", IFIP-68.

Childs, D.L. (1968b) "Description of a set-theoretical data structure", AFIPS 1968.

Childs, D.L. (1974) "Extended Set Theory" STIS Corp.

CODASYL (1962) "An information algebra", CACM, 5, 190-204.

CODASYL (1971) "Data base task group report", ACM, New York.

Codd, E.F. (1970) "A relational model of data for large shared data banks", CACM 13, pp. 377-387.

Codd, E.F. (1971a) "Further normalization of the data base relational model", Data Base Systems ed. by R. Rustin.

Codd, E.F. (1971b) "Relational completeness of data base sublanguages", Data Base Systems ed. by R. Rustin.

Debeneffe, C., Heunebert, H. and Paulus, W. (1974) "Relational model for a data base", Proc. IFIP-74, North Holland, 1974.

Durchholz, R. and Richter, G. (1974) "Concepts for data base management systems", Data Base Management, J.W. Klimbie and K.L. Koffeman (eds.), North Holland, 1974.

Durchholz, R. and Richter, G. (1976) "Information management concepts (IMC) for use with DBMS interface", Proc. IFIP-TC-2-WC, Black Forest.

Fillmore, C. (1968) "The case for case", Universals in Linguistic Theory, E. Bach and R. Harms (eds.), Holt, Rinehart and Winston, 1968.

Hall, P., Owlett, J. and Todd, S. (1976) "Relations and Entities", Proc. IFIP-TC-2-WC, Black Forest.

Kerschberg, L. and Pacheco, J.E.S. (1975) "A functional data base model", monograph, Pontificia Universidade Catolica do Rio de Janeiro, 1975.

Kobayashi, I. (1975) "Information and information processing structure", Information Systems 1, pp. 39-49.

Langefors, B. (1966) "Theoretical Analysis of Information Systems", Studentlitterature, Lund, Sweden, 1966.

Langefors, B. (1974) "Information Systems", Proc. IFIP-74, North Holland, 1974.

Leech, G. (1974) "Semantics", Penguin Books Ltd., Middlesex, England, 1974.

Lindgreen, P. (1974) "Basic operations on information as a basis for data base design", Proc. IFIP-74, North Holland, 1974.

Moulin, P., Randon, J., Teboul, M., u.a. (1976) "Conceptual model as a data base design tool", Proc. IFIP-TC-2-WC, Black Forest.

Mylopoulos, J. et al. (1975) "The TORUS project: progress report", Department of Computer Science, University of Toronto.

Nijssen, G.M. (1975) "Set and CODASYL set or coset", Data Base Description, Douque and Nijssen (eds.), North Holland, 1975.

Roussopoulos, N. and Mylopoulos, J. (1975) "Using semantic networks for data base management", Conf. on V.L.D.B.

Schmid, H.A. and Swenson, J.R. (1975) "On the semantics of the relational data model", ACM SIGMOD-75.

Senko, M.E., Altman, E.B., Astrahan, M.M. and Fehder, P.L. (1973) "Data structures and accessing in data-base systems", IBM Systems J. 1973, pp. 30-93.

Senko, M.E., (1975) "Specification of stored data structures and desired output results in DIAM-II with FORAL", Conf. on V.L.D.B. 1975.

Steel, T.B. (1975) "Data base standardization: a status report", Data Base Description, Douque and Nijssen (eds.), North Holland, 1975.

Sundgren, B. (1974) "Conceptual foundation of the infological approach to data bases", Data Base Management, J.W. Klimbie and K.L.Koffeman (eds.), North Holland, 1974.

Tsichritzis, D.C. (1975) "Features of a conceptual schema", Conf. on V.I.D.B. 1975 and CSRG-56, University of Toronto.

Tsichritzis, D.C. (1975b) "LSL - a link and selector language", ACM SIGMOD-76.

*Systems for Large Data Bases, P.C. Lockemann and E.J. Neuhold, (eds.)*
*North-Holland Publishing Company, 1976*

# CHOOSING AN EFFICIENT INTERNAL SCHEMA

Frank Wm. Tompa
Department of Computer Science
University of Waterloo
Waterloo, Ontario, Canada
N2L 3G1

The internal schema for a data base should not be concocted in an ad hoc manner, but rather result from an algorithmic design. This paper describes a methodology for choosing an efficient internal schema for a data base, given the conceptual schema and a target machine. It is assumed that the conceptual schema is composed of abstract data types which have associated "activity profiles" reflecting expected usage (e.g., expected set sizes and relative frequencies for insertions and deletions).

The methodology requires the construction of a library of permissible realizations for each abstract data type which may be used in any conceptual schema. Each member of the library is a *cluster* of code implementing the defined operations for one particular representation of a data type. (These clusters, which are invoked when a program accesses a data base, may be regarded as either open or closed subroutines.) Using the target machine's functional characteristics, a translator compiling the code can automatically generate parametric formulas which represent the expected run time and storage space used by the data that is to be manipulated by each cluster.

The application of the methodology itself starts with the construction of an evaluation matrix, for which the entries are derived from the library's parametric formulas by substituting values which reflect each component of the conceptual schema. Thus, for every occurrence of a data type in the conceptual schema, this matrix incorporates the expected run time and storage space required for each cluster which may be used to realize that type. The evaluation matrix is then searched using branch and bound to choose, for each data type occurrence, that cluster which minimizes the internal schema's overall cost.

The major advantage of this approach is that it includes a comparison of all internal representations which can be realized by superimposing members from a library. Therefore, a cluster which is traditionally used in one specific application, and which is therefore present in the library, will be considered for every occurrence of the corresponding type in the conceptual schema. Automation of the algorithm results in a thorough, yet efficient, evaluation of all alternatives, thus ensuring an efficient data base representation.

KEY PHRASES

mapping from a conceptual schema to an internal schema, efficiency of storage structures, space-time trade-off.

## INTRODUCTION

Many data base designers have agreed that data should be viewed at three separate levels [ANSI(1976)]: the external schema which incorporates one user's view, the conceptual schema which integrates all users' views, and the internal schema which reflects the storage structure (the "machine view"). Although data base design involves a great deal of insight and artistry by the designers, there are parts which can be made algorithmic. In particular, an internal schema which will be an efficient representation for a given conceptual schema can be chosen automatically.

The major difficulty in designing an internal schema is that the number of possible representations for a complex data base is too large to examine with care. To reduce the complexity, the efficiency of simple structures can be evaluated first, and then, using these evaluations, the costs of internal schemata produced by superimposing these representations can be compared. Although the number of choices for representing a simple relation (e.g., a single data type such as an array, a sequence, or a set) is much smaller than the number which can represent a composite internal schema, even for a single data type many representations have been described in the literature, and many more could still be described.

## THE LIBRARY OF STORAGE STRUCTURES

To evaluate all possible representations for a data type would be extremely inefficient, if not impossible. In addition, there seems to be no ordering of the representations which would enable an efficient evaluation that involves the whole space of representations.

The approach adopted here is to consider only representations available from a given library. To contain representations used in current applications, this library would likely include contiguous tables, hash tables, linear linked lists, and a variety of tree structures [Gotlieb(1974), Yao(1975)]. In practice for applications using a data manipulation language, the library would consist of those representations which can be generated by the language's translator. To choose an optimal internal schema is not the goal here, but rather to choose one which is the most efficient implementation as generated by the data base translator.

In general, a conceptual schema may contain several data types (e.g., record, repeating group, numeric, string) each of which has a set of defined operations (e.g., GET NEXT, INSERT, REPLACE, AVERAGE). For each data type, the library should contain one or more clusters of code which implement the operations for that type [cf. Dahl(1968), Liskov(1974)]. Furthermore, since the choice of representations will depend on the efficiency of the implementation, it would be convenient for each data type to have an associated costs table. For each potential representation for the data type, this table should contain an entry indicating formulas for expected run time and storage space in terms of parameters which will reflect the role of the data type in the conceptual schema. For example, the parametric table entries for a repeating group would likely contain formulas for representations by contiguous storage and by a singly-linked list. These formulas, expressed in terms of the expected number of elements in the group; the expected size of each element; the expected target position for a retrieval request (e.g., whether all requests are at the start or, instead, uniformly distributed over the group); and the expected number of insertions, deletions, and traversals, may then be evaluated in light of an application's parametric values as determined from the algorithms used on the conceptual schema (i.e., as mapped from the many external schemata).

At least two systems have been described for parameterizing the expected run time for a program. In one [Cohen(1974a)], a program written in a language similar to Algol 60 is translated into a LISP structure in which each source-level construct is replaced by an expression that parametrically represents the time to execute that program. In the other [Tompa(1974)], a language was designed with a syntax in which every symbol in a program has an associated run time, and the expected time for a complete program can be determined easily during parsing. Using a similar system which models a multi-level store, the basic operations defined for each data type may be encoded. Thus the run time for each representation in the library can be determined with respect to parameters which represent how many times each function is executed, as well as how many times loops are executed, whether conditions will be true or false, and the timing characteristics of the hardware. The resulting formulas form the run time entries in the parametric table for that data type.

Unlike the evaluation of run time, the measurement of storage space is not directly dependent on the processes involved in the application. In fact, the amount of storage space at each storage level can be specified as a function of

- the number of occurring elements,
- the maximum number of elements likely to occur at any one time,
- the number of possible elements,
- the number of cells per element, and
- the size of each cell.*

Therefore, parametric formulas which represent the storage space can also be entered into the tables.

## USING AN EVALUATION MATRIX TO CHOOSE AN INTERNAL SCHEMA

To choose an internal schema for a given conceptual schema, the latter must first be described in terms of *substructures*, each of which is an instance of a data type for which an implementation choice is to be made [Gotlieb(1974)]. For example, if a student record file consists of arbitrarily many student records, each of which has fields for course number and course name, and repeating groups for meeting times and grades, (assuming the implementation for fields to be fixed) the file will be said to have four substructures: the file itself, each individual record, the repeating group for times, and the repeating group for grades.

---

* The possibility of overlapping clusters to share data complicates the analysis of storage space requirements. The user must supply additional semantic information to allow the system to consider shared data. The problem can be circumvented by assuming that the parametric values have been adjusted by the user such that each item of data is reflected once only.

Next, for each substructure, the library's parametric table corresponding to the substructure's data type must be evaluated by substituting parametric values that reflect the substructure's role within the conceptual schema. These calculations will each produce a column of an evaluation matrix, such that the element pair in row i and column j represents the run time and storage space contributed by the j-th substructure when represented by the i-th cluster in the library.*

The calculation of expected run time is straightforward. For the algorithms on the conceptual schema (as translated from the external schemata), the values of most of a cluster's parameters can be determined, the rest being assigned default values. These values are then substituted into the time formula for the cluster, yielding the expected run time (in microseconds), which is then assigned to the appropriate component of the evaluation matrix.

The space required by a substructure is the product of the number of cells used by the cluster representing that substructure, and the number of copies of that substructure in the application. Thus, for example, the space required by a cluster representing a student record must be multiplied by the number of student records in the file. If this product were entered into the matrix, however, the space used by a dependent substructure (one wholly contained within another) may be represented twice: first as the dependent substructure itself, and second as a set of fields within one of the member elements of the substructure on which it depends. For the student record example, the space charged for the repeating group of meeting times in each record should not include the space already charged as part of the student record itself. To avoid this duplication, it is necessary to count only the number of cells for that part of each substructure which would be located outside all other substructures for multiplying by the expected number of instances. The space entry will therefore contain that product (henceforth called the separate space) separately from the space which will lie within another substructure (the nested space).**

Given such an evaluation matrix and a user-supplied cost formula as a function of space and/or time, a cluster may be assigned to each substructure such that the resulting composite internal schema has minimal cost over all such cluster assignments. Unfortunately, in general, the least cost for the whole application is not achieved when each substructure uses the least-cost cluster. For example, consider an application having the evaluation matrix shown in Figure 1a, in which, for simplicity, only one space entry per matrix element is shown. For the cost formula represented by space*time, a matrix of costs could be derived by evaluating each element individually (Figure 1b).

---

* The orderings of the substructures and the library's members do not affect the evaluation's outcome, but they may affect the efficiency of the evaluation itself.

** Where programs and data are allocated storage from the same memory, the space required for manipulation routines can also be entered into the matrix separately.

Figure 1 MISUSING AN EVALUATION MATRIX

| | | substructures 1 | substructures 2 |
|---|---|---|---|
| clusters | 1 | (50 cells, 50 msec.) | (1 cell, 100 msec.) |
| | 2 | (100 cells, 1 msec.) | (40 cells, 60 msec.) |

a) A simplified evaluation matrix

| | | substructures 1 | substructures 2 |
|---|---|---|---|
| clusters | 1 | 2500 cell-msec. | 100 cell-msec. |
| | 2 | 100 cell-msec. | 2400 cell-msec. |

b) The corresponding matrix of costs.

From Figure 1b, it seems that cluster 2 has the least cost for substructure 1, and cluster 1 has least cost for substructure 2. However, since the cost is total space times total time, using these assignments to implement the application would result in a cost of (100+1 cells) * (1+100 msec.) = 10201 cell-msec. This is clearly not minimal: using the first cluster for both substructures would result in a lesser cost, namely (50+1 cells) * (50+100 msec.) = 7650 cell-msec.

Because choosing the cluster of least cost for each substructure will not guarantee an efficient internal schema, it would seem at first that all possible combinations of clusters must be examined. This is impractical for large applications, however, because the number of cluster assignments grows exponentially in the number of substructures. Therefore, a technique must be adopted for reducing the expected number which need to be evaluated explicitly.

Branch and bound, which has been used successfully in many areas of operations research, can be applied to direct the search for an efficient storage structure. "The space of all feasible solutions is repeatedly partitioned into smaller and smaller subsets, and a lower bound ... is calculated for the cost of the solutions within each subset. After each partitioning, those subsets with a bound that exceeds the cost of a known feasible solution are excluded from all further partitioning" [Lawler(1966)].

Applied to this algorithm, the branching phase partitions sets of potential internal schemata by considering one substructure at a time. Consider, for example, an application consisting of three substructures, each of which can be represented by any of four clusters (thus there are $4^3 = 64$ potential representations). The set of all potential internal schemata can be partitioned along the first substructure into four subsets: those in which the first substructure is represented by cluster 1, by cluster 2, by cluster 3 and by cluster 4, respectively. It is convenient to represent the state of cluster assignments by an assignment vector in which each position corresponds to a substructure and each non-null entry corresponds to the number of the cluster assigned. For example, the initial assignment vector would be (,,), indicating that any cluster may be used for any substructure. After branching along the first substructure, four new assignment vectors would be generated (1,,), (2,,), (3,,), and (4,,). Choosing the second set of potential internal schemata for subsequent branching would result in four new subsets, represented by (2,1,), (2,2,), (2,3,), and (2,4,). Finally partitioning the first of these would produce four fully-defined representations (2,1,1), (2,1,2), (2,1,3), and (2,1,4). The complete branching into subsets can be illustrated in the form of a tree of assignment vectors (Figure 2).

Figure 2 BRANCHING OF A SET OF STORAGE STRUCTURES INTO SUBSETS

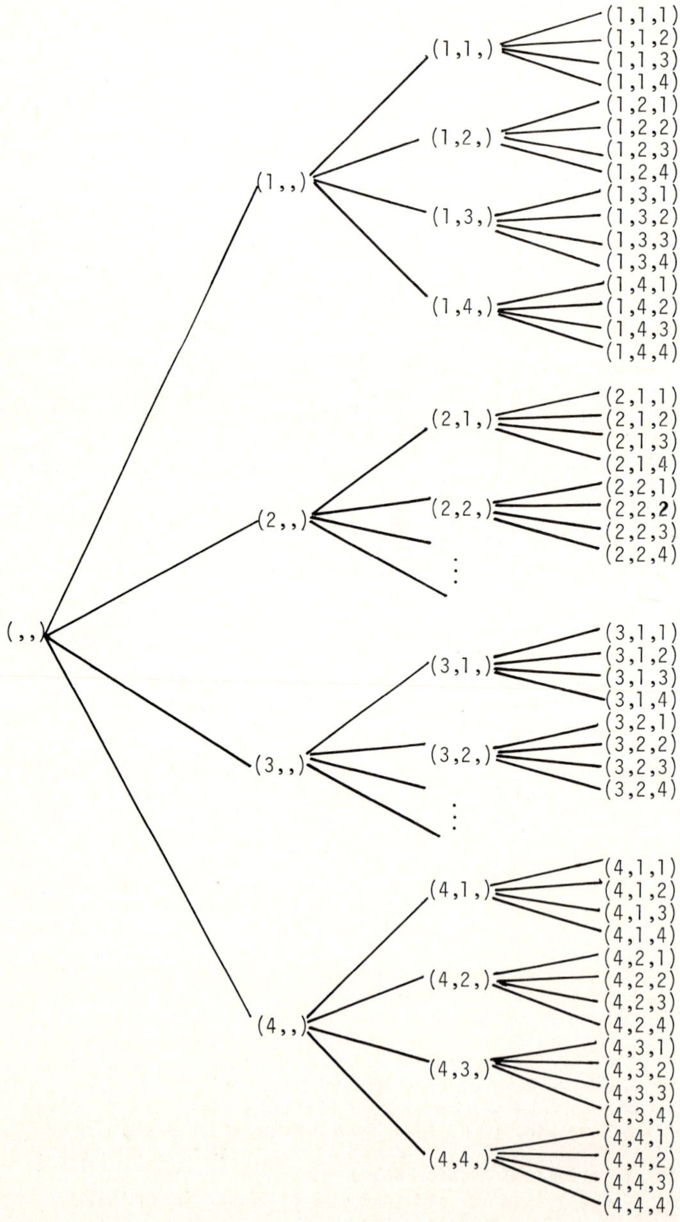

Because the clusters are to be superimposed in a given machine, and not only in a mathematical model, the characteristics of the machine must be considered in order to avoid any contention (e.g., for limited memory space) [Gotlieb(1974)]. Thus, given an assignment vector, v, and a substructure, j, for which v(j) = null, a preliminary pruning phase must be invoked to eliminate those clusters which would lead to contention if assigned to the j-th substructure. That phase can further reduce the number of possible cluster assignments for v(j) by eliminating those for which the cost for performing a needed operation is prohibitive (e.g., an implementation requiring a complete scan of memory).

The branching of a set of cluster assignments, represented by vector v, into subsets is therefore accomplished as follows:

- Find the index of the first null entry, J.
- Use the preliminary pruning phase to eliminate all clusters which cannot be chosen for the J-th substructure.
- For each of the k clusters $i_J^1,\ldots,i_J^k$ remaining in the library, create a new assignment vector $v^I$ such that $v^I(j) = v(j)$ for $j \neq J$, and $v^I(j) = i_J^I$.

If the set of all potential internal schemata were to be fully partitioned, as implied by Figure 2, and each node of the tree were to be evaluated, the cost for evaluation would still grow exponentially. It is the second stage of branch and bound which attempts to prune the tree by finding lower bounds on cost for all members of designated subsets. For example, if a lower bound on cost for the representations in the set represented by assignment vector (1,,) were found to be greater than the cost for the internal schema represented by (2,1,3), there would be no need to evaluate the top quarter of the tree in Figure 2. When (as usual) the cost formula, F, is a non-decreasing function of run time and storage space, one lower bound on cost for the members of a set is the value of F applied to the fastest possible time for that set and the smallest possible space for that set (which are not necessarily simultaneously achievable).

To calculate the fastest possible time for a set of assignments v, a temporary assignment vector Tv is constructed, in which if v(j) ≠ null, Tv(j) is set to v(j), and if v(j) = null, Tv(j) is set to the index of the cluster requiring least time after pruning. (If several clusters have the same minimal time, one of those with least space should be chosen for Tv(j).) It is important that, for each substructure, the library is pruned with respect to v, rather than to that part of Tv which has already been constructed, in order that the clusters are chosen independently for all null entries in v. The least time for v, t(v), is the sum of the run times for the components of Tv.

To calculate the least possible space for v, a second temporary vector Sv is constructed similarly, except that Sv(j) is set to the index of the cluster requiring least *space* for the member elements after pruning for each of the null entries in v. The total space for a component of Sv must include the cells required for the *nested space of any dependent substructures* if and only if the index in v for that dependent substructure is not null; otherwise, the value for the smallest possible nested space should be used in place of the nested space for that component. Furthermore, for a substructure which is *not* contained within any others, the value for its *own* nested space must be added, regardless of the null entries in v. The least space for v, s(v), is then the sum of the space required for the components of Sv.

The lower bound on cost for v, denoted c(v), is therefore F(t(v),s(v)). If (1) Tv = Sv, (2) each null entry in v which corresponds to a dependent substructure has been assigned a cluster in which the nested space is minimal in size, *and* (3) all the clusters represented in Tv happen to be free from contention, then the internal schema designated by Tv is a feasible solution for which the cost therefore provides an upper bound for the application. It is this upper bound which is used to eliminate sets of representations having greater lower bounds on cost.

The complete algorithm for searching an evaluation matrix is thus illustrated in Figure 3. The algorithm, given an evaluation matrix and a cost formula, returns the assignment vector and cost for the most efficient internal schema.

## AN EXAMPLE OF INTERNAL SCHEMA DESIGN

The methodology will be illustrated by designing the internal schema for a system for natural language understanding [Cohen(1974b)]. In that system, English syntax and semantics were modelled by a labeled, directed graph on which the following processes were defined:

P1. Determine whether there is an edge beginning and ending at given nodes (hereafter called the source node and target node, respectively), such that the edge has a given label.

P2. Find a target node, given a source node and an edge label.

P3. Find a source node, given a target node and an edge label.

P4. Add a labeled edge between two (not necessarily distinct) given nodes.

P5. Delete a given edge between two given nodes.

P6. Add a node to the graph.

P7. Delete a node from the graph, and delete all edges to and from that node.

Expected usage of the graphs led the designers to define the conceptual schema as follows:

```
type graph = set of node;
type node = (set of node PREDECESSORS;
             set of edge_class OUT_EDGES);
type edge_class = (string LABEL; set of node SUCCESSORS)
```

This choice determined the algorithms which could be used to manipulate the data base. For example, finding the set of nodes *adjacent to node N* via an edge labeled E (process P2) implied scanning the set OUT_EDGES(N) for an edge_class which has LABEL E and returning the corresponding SUCCESSORS. On the other hand, finding the set of nodes *to which node N is adjacent* via an edge labeled E (process P3) implied traversing the set PREDECESSORS(N) for nodes that have an edge_class with LABEL E and with SUCCESSORS including N. The following Algol-like procedures encode these algorithms at the level of the conceptual schema:

Figure 3 ALGORITHM FOR SEARCHING AN EVALUATION MATRIX

```
Determine Tv, Sv, and c(v^0) for v^0, the assignment vector having
   null entries only
If Tv is a feasible solution
   Then Set Choice to the pair <Tv,c(v^0)>
   Else Initialize Choice with the pair <null, infinite cost>
        Initialize S, a set of vectors to consider, with the
           ordered pair <v^0,c(v^0)>  as its only member
        While S is not empty:
           Choose the assignment vector, V in S, with least c(V)
              and delete the corresponding ordered pair from S
           Apply the branching to V to obtain new vectors, V'
           For each of the V':
              Determine Tv, Sv, and c(V')
              If c(V') is less than the cost for Choice
                 Then If Tv is a feasible solution
                         Then Replace Choice by <Tv,c(V')>
                              For each ordered pair <v,c(v)> in S
                                 If c(v) > c(V')
                                    Then Delete the pair from S
                                 end "For each" loop
                         Else Add <V',c(V')> to S
              end "For each" loop
           end "While" loop
If the cost of Choice is finite
   Then The assignment vector chosen has minimal cost
   Else There is no solution for the application
```

```
(set of node) procedure SUCCESSOR (node N; string E);
          begin
          set of node S;
          S := empty;
          for I ∈ OUT_EDGES(N) do
             if LABEL(I) = E
                then S := SUCCESSORS(I);
          S
          end;
(set of node) procedure PREDECESSOR (node N; string E);
          begin
          set of node S;
          S := empty;
          for P ∈ PREDECESSORS(N) do
              for I ∈ OUT_EDGES(P) do
                  if LABEL(I) = E
                      then if N ∈ SUCCESSORS(I)
                              then S := S ∪ {P};
          S
          end
```

Similarly, for each process, an algorithm was written in terms of the operations defined on the data types involved (i.e. sets).

The next step in the design process is to determine the values for the parameters appearing in the library's tables, which for the example will be assumed to contain formulas for fifteen clusters for representing sets. For representing a short English-language discourse it may be assumed that there are approximately 100 nodes, an average of 5 edge labels per node, 1.5 target nodes per edge label, and 4 predecessors per node. Furthermore, it will be assumed that there is exactly one loop on each node (specifying the "name" of that node), and 25 distinct labels appearing on edges between pairs of nodes anywhere in the graph. Finally, the relative frequencies of invoking P1 through P7 is estimated to be 25%, 20%, 20%, 10%, 10%, 5%, and respectively.*

This presentation will by-pass choosing a cluster for the first substructure, the set of nodes. For reasons which are superfluous to the illustration, it will be assumed that that substructure will be represented by the second cluster in the library; thus $v^0$, the initial vector for the algorithm, is (2,,,).

Figure 4 illustrates the evaluation matrix for this application, in which the run times represent the expected time for any <u>one</u> invocation of a process. When the branch and bound method is invoked, Tv and Sv must first be calculated for $v^0$. From Figure 4 it can be seen that Tv = (2,2,6,2) and the Sv = (2,11,11,11). Since the system was designed to be used at the University of Toronto, that university's charging algorithm will be assumed; thus,

$$F(s,t) = (1.42*10^{-7})t + (.7*10^{-10})t*s + (.56*10^{-18})t*s^2$$

where t is in microseconds and s is in cells (which are assumed to be four bytes each). Therefore, assuming that data manipulation dominates all operations, the lower bound on cost is $c(v^0) = \$.99*10^{-4}$ for each process invocation. Since Tv ≠ Sv, Tv is not a feasible solution, and the branch and bound algorithm proceeds to search the matrix.

---

* The expected values were estimated by P. Cohen and L. Melli from their experience with the natural language understanding system.

Figure 4 EVALUATION MATRIX FOR COHEN'S SYSTEM

Substructure 1 is to be implemented using the second cluster: thus the single matrix entry required is (33, (2,3) ).

| | Substructure 2 | | | Substructure 3 | | | Substructure 4 | | |
|---|---|---|---|---|---|---|---|---|---|
| | | space | | | space | | | space | |
| cluster | time | separate | nested | time | separate | nested | time | separate | nested |
| 1 | 186.6 | 15 | 3 | 134.3 | 22.5 | 3 | 81.6 | 12 | 3 |
| 2 | 156.7 | 15 | 3 | 127.6 | 22.5 | 3 | 73.5 | 12 | 3 |
| 3 | 190.9 | 20 | 4 | 213.3 | 30 | 4 | 104.1 | 16 | 4 |
| 4 | 157.7 | 20 | 4 | 131.3 | 30 | 4 | 74.3 | 16 | 4 |
| 5 | ∞ | 10 | 2 | ∞ | 15 | 2 | ∞ | 8 | 2 |
| 6 | 161.4 | 10 | 2 | 124.3 | 15 | 2 | 75.3 | 8 | 2 |
| 7 | ∞ | 15 | 3 | ∞ | 22.5 | 3 | ∞ | 12 | 3 |
| 8 | 323.2 | 20 | 4 | 264.4 | 30 | 4 | 148.8 | 16 | 4 |
| 9 | ∞ | 25 | 5 | ∞ | 37.5 | 5 | ∞ | 20 | 5 |
| 10 | 320.8 | 25 | 5 | 267.2 | 37.5 | 5 | 153.1 | 20 | 5 |
| 11 | 274.9 | 0 | 23 | 153.9 | 0 | 7 | 100.8 | 0 | 27 |
| 12 | 736.5 | 0 | 23 | 409.3 | 0 | 7 | 677.1 | 0 | 27 |
| 13 | ∞ | 0 | ∞ | ∞ | 0 | ∞ | ∞ | 0 | ∞ |
| 14 | ∞ | 5 | 14 | ∞ | 7.5 | 9 | ∞ | 4 | 29 |
| 15 | ∞ | 15 | 3 | ∞ | 22.5 | 3 | ∞ | 12 | 3 |

N.B. Time is in microseconds and space is in cells (which are assumed to be four bytes each).

After finding the costs of 73 assignment vectors (which represent 729 potential storage structures having finite cost), the algorithm terminates producing the vector (2,6,6,6) and a cost of $1.91*10^{-4}$ for each process invocation.* This choice represents a 14% improvement in run time over the internal schema originally designed and adopted for the data base. Unfortunately, the actual cost reduction is only 4% because of an increase in storage space.

After reconsidering the conceptual schema in light of insights provided by using this algorithm, it was redesigned to consist of three substructures only: a set of labeled nodes, a set of out-edges for each node (i.e., edges for which the node is a source), and a set of in-edges for each node (i.e., edges for which the node is a target). That is,

```
type graph = set of node;
type node = (set of edge OUT_EDGES, IN_EDGES);
type edge = (string LABEL; node ADJACENT);
```

This revision requires new algorithms to be written for the processes. Again an evaluation matrix can be constructed using the new parametric values, and the branch and bound algorithm can be invoked to find the best representation. The cluster assignment which results is (2,6,6), for which the cost is only $1.66*10^{-4}$ per process invocation. This represents at 16% *cost* reduction with respect to the data base's original design.

## CONCLUSIONS

This paper presents a procedure for choosing an internal schema which will be efficient for a given conceptual schema. The algorithmic approach to choosing an internal schema is superior to intuitive methodologies in several respects. Foremost, the algorithm includes a comparison of all structures which can be realized by superimposing components from a library. Therefore, a cluster which is traditionally used in one specific application, and which is therefore included in the library, will be considered for any substructure having the same data type. Although the resulting choice may not be counter-intuitive, it is often not what intuition would dictate.

A second aspect favouring the algorithm is its speed. Because of the parametric approach, the evaluation matrix entries for each substructure can be calculated quickly. While it is true that searching the matrix may require an amount of time that grows exponentially in the number of substructures, the branch and bound technique is a systematic search which attempts to eliminate many potential computations. Furthermore, there have been several heuristics suggested for increasing the efficiency in branch and bound searches, including methods for computing suboptimal solutions [Lawler(1966)]. Additional improvement in the algorithm's speed can be obtained by judiciously ordering the substructures (matrix columns), such that the substructures having the least number of choices and the "clearest" choice of clusters occur first. (In this way, the exponentiality of the search will be reduced.) Therefore, unlike traditional hand analyses, the method is fast enough to allow many alternatives to be considered.

---

* The sixth cluster represents sets as singly-linked rings in which member elements are ordered by value and the owner element contains a "dummy value" which is greater than any member's value.

## ACKNOWLEDGEMENTS

Thanks are due to C.C. Gotlieb for his help in formulating these ideas, and to P. Cohen for his donation of the natural language understanding system. Acknowledgement is also given to the University of Toronto, The University of Waterloo, and to the National Research Council of Canada for their financial support.

## REFERENCES

ANSI/X3/SPARC study group on data base management systems (1975), Interim report 75-02-08. *FDT 7*, 2, pp. 1-140.

J. Cohen and C. Zuckerman (June 1974), Two languages for estimating program efficiency, *Comm. ACM 17*, 6, pp. 301-308.

P.R. Cohen (March 1974), A prototype natural language understanding system. Department of Computer Science, University of Toronto, Tech. Report 64, pp. 1-149.

O.J. Dahl, K. Nygaard, and B. Myhrhuag (1968), The SIMULA 67 common base language. Norwegian Computing Centre, Forskningsveien 1B, Oslo.

C.C. Gotlieb and F.W. Tompa (1974), Choosing a storage schema. *Acta Informatica 3*, pp. 297-319.

E.L. Lawler and D.E. Wood (1966), Branch and bound methods: a survey. *Op. Res. 14*, 4, pp. 699-719.

B. Liskov and S. Zilles (April 1974), Programming with abstract data types. *Proc. of a Symp. on Very High Level Languages. SIGPLAN NOTICES 9*, 4, pp. 50-59.

F.W. Tompa (1974), Choosing a data storage schema. Ph.D. thesis, Department of Computer Science, University of Toronto, pp. 1-241.

S.B. Yao and A.G. Merten (Sept. 1975), Selection of file organization using an analytic model. *Proc. of the Int. Conf. on Very Large Data Bases*, D.S. Kerr, ed., pp. 255-267.

*Systems for Large Data Bases, P.C. Lockemann and E.J. Neuhold, (eds.)*
*North-Holland Publishing Company, 1976*

# DIAM II and Levels of Abstraction

# The Physical Device Level:

# A General Model for Access Methods

Michael E. Senko

Mathematical Sciences Department
IBM Thomas J. Watson Research Center
Yorktown Heights, New York

Edward B. Altman

Systems Performance Evaluation Department
IBM General Products Division
Palo Alto, California

At present, levels of abstraction are being used as a major tool for discussing, simplifying, clarifying, and improving data base systems. In the data base area, this level strategy has a history which includes notable early papers of Madnick (1) and Meltzer (2). In such early papers, the components of the abstract levels were pragmatically extracted from existing systems. Recent papers are using more formal components.

For example, the initial Data Independent Accessing Model, DIAM I, (3) gave a detailed formal basis - a set of components and mappings - for four abstract levels. At its Entity Set Level (the abstract level that was its data structure independent view of the real world), DIAM I followed Meltzer (2) and Mealy in emphasizing the semantic nature of the level's components and their associations.

More recently, the ANSI SPARC Committee (5) has defined a structure containing three major abstract levels. This group gave increased stature to an *External Schema Level* above the four DIAM levels. It also gave clear recognition to the requirements for a canonical, data independent *Conceptual Level* which corresponds closely in function to DIAM I's Entity Set Level. The third ANSI level, the *Internal Model*, contains the other three DIAM levels, (a) an access path level, (b) an encoding level, and (c) a physical device level.

This ANSI work on levels, along with the earlier work of Levien and Maron (6), Langefors (7), Sundgren (8), and Abrial (9) on binary representations has been used to modify and improve the original DIAM. The resulting DIAM II (10, 11, 12) contains an *End-User Level* (ANSI External Schema Level) and a canonical *Infological Level* (ANSI Conceptual Schema) based on modified binary associations. This latter level provides a fundamental improvement in semantic integrity over the Entity Set Model of DIAM I and the somewhat similar n-ary relational model.

The DIAM II End-User and Infological Levels with their accessing language (FORAL), as well as the adjacent two internal levels (the access path and encoding levels) have been discussed elsewhere. Their characteristics will only be summarized in this paper. We now complete a detailed discussion of the abstract levels in DIAM with this paper on the Physical Device Level. At this level, DIAM uses three basic building blocks, Address Spaces, Internal Records and Frames, to provide a general model of access methods.

## THE GENERAL LEVEL STRUCTURE OF DIAM II

In Figure 1, we present the DIAM II "Double Funnel" diagram. The funnels opening upward and downward indicate that the system supports a wider variety of data structures at its upper and lower levels than it does at its canonical Infological Level.

The upper End-User Level is designed to support many (possibly redundant) data structure views. These views are designed to provide both end-user efficiency and compatibility with the data structures of existing programming languages (FORTRAN, COBOL, DBTG, IMS, etc.). Similarly the three internal datalogical levels provide a general set of file organizations to support efficient use of the computer. The Infological level, in agreement with ANSI SPARC requirements, is designed to be canonical in its representation of the user's enterprise.

In Figure 2, we present an example view of the binary association *Infological Level* of DIAM II.

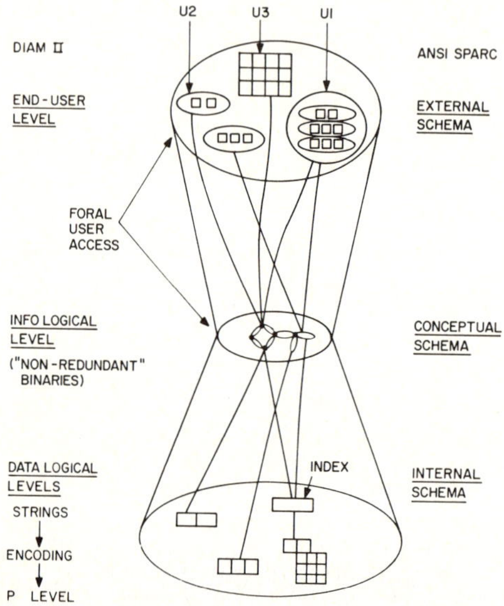


Figure 1 DIAM II - ANSI SPARC System Overviews

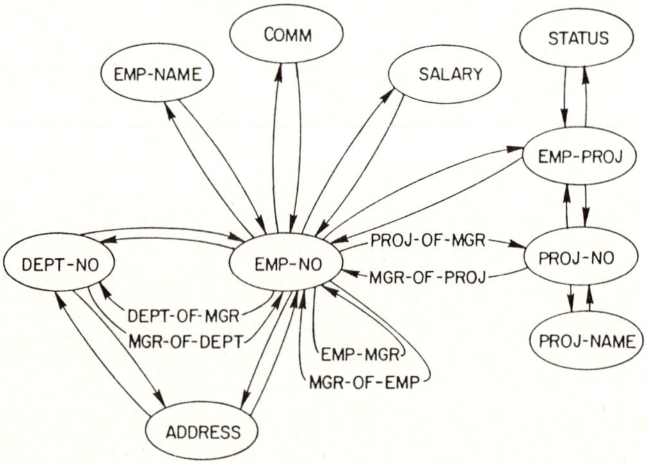


Figure 2 DIAM Infological Level

The ovals (containing EMP-NO, DEPT-NO, etc.) stand for lists of names for important entities. (In an alternate representation, they can stand instead for sets of entities.) An arrow pointing from one oval to a second oval (for example, from EMP-NO to DEPT-NO) indicates that the second oval gives attribute values for the first.

These arrows represent the only meaningful direct associations between entities in the system.

The FORAL language, by limiting the user to statements that traverse attribute arrows one at a time, allows him to state only transactions that make semantic sense in terms of his information structure. A typical FORAL II statement might be:

```
output MY-OUTPUT:
EMP-NO
    (where SALARY greater-than 30)
for DEPT-NO
    print
    MGR-OF-DEPT.
```

MY-OUTPUT would contain the EMP-NO of each employee (with SALARY greater than 30), and for his DEPT-NO, the MGR-OF-DEPT.

The DIAM II *Access Path Level* is based on ordered subsets of information elements from the Infological Level. It is a general model for specifying efficient access paths for user transactions.

There are two kinds of strings in DIAM II: Instance Strings and Type Strings. The Instance Strings give direct access to a specified ordered subset of the attribute values of a particular entity. For example, an I-String might connect EMP-NO, 12345 with his attributes, NAME, SALARY, and DEPT-NO. An I-String is something like a single level record.

A Type-String connects subsets of instances of the same type. For example, a T-String might connect together all the members of DEPT-NO, 420. Combinations of these two primitive kinds of strings may be defined to provide the user with the access path equivalents of most file organization elements (secondary indexes, hierarchic records, generation data groups, etc.)

The next lower level in DIAM is the *Encoding Level*. This level provides a generalized model for specifying bit encodings of access path nodes.

The primitive element of this level is the Basic Encoding Unit (BEU). There is one type of BEU for each type of string and one BEU instance for each instance of an attribute value or string. The parameters defined for the BEU allow the user to specify anything from a generalized list structure to a completely contiguous grouping of data elements. In DIAM I, these contiguous groups of data elements were called Contiguous Data Groups (CDG's). They correspond to ANSI SPARC "Internal Records".

Much work has been published on data independent levels corresponding to the DIAM Infological Level. This work is important, but it has avoided responsibility for solution of the more difficult and challenging computer efficiency problem. The data independent models will only see widespread usage when this latter problem is reasonably well solved.

DIAM's attack on the computer efficiency problem begins with its general model for defining efficient access paths. Other literature is only now beginning to appear on alternate definitions of access paths (Manacher (13), Schmid and Bernstein (14), and Tsichritzis (16)). In most cases, the access structures in their work seem to be a subset of the DIAM access path level.

Although works on data translation like that of Smith (17) attack the encoding problem at a microscopic, bit level, very little, other than the DIAM work, has been done on a level for generalized encoding.

The final level that is needed to complete the efficient mapping of an infological level to actual devices is one that provides the functions of access methods. Only Hsiao and Harary (16), Smith (17) and Taylor and Sibley (18) seem to have worked on generalized models for this level. These models either cover a limited set of functions or are exceedingly detailed in their specifications. Another model based on DIAM principles, using the top three levels of DIAM I, has recently been published by L. Schneider (19).

The generalized access method model in this paper is based on an earlier IBM Research Report by Senko and Altman (20). It covers a wide range of complex access methods with a generalized parameterization of three basic building blocks.

## THE DIAM PHYSICAL DEVICE LEVEL

In DIAM, the Physical Device Level manages storage of Internal Records. (Since we will only be discussing Internal Records in this paper, we will use the term, Record, as a shorthand.)

There are at least two reasons for managing storage of records.

(a) A desire to keep records in order so merges, sorts, large file comparisons, etc. can be performed efficiently.

(b) A desire to cluster the records for a particular query in a small physical area to minimize page faults.

The challenge for record management is to provide these properties with performance and efficiency in the face of unpredictable kinds of record insertions.

### Possible Solutions

There are numerous specific access methods, each with its specific set of desirable properties. The problem is that any single access method lacks many desirable functions. The normal, brute force way to overcome these shortcomings is to provide a set of overlapping, inconsistent access methods, each with a significant amount of redundant function and program coding. To simplify the situation, it would be desirable to provide all the desired functions in a systematic consistent manner.

In the following sections, we will use the three basic building blocks: *Address Spaces*, *Records*, and *Frames* along with recursion of these concepts to equip DIAM with an access method level capable of providing the desirable properties a simple, coherent fashion. Different access method properties can then be obtained by simply changing a few paramenter values. There will be no need to write a considerable amount of new redundant code.

We will start our discussion of desirable functions with simple, restricted examples of record handling. We will then gradually move to the general model. As in the discussion of the DIAM Basic Encoding Unit, we will present a precise parameterization of the basic building blocks. Finally, we will discuss a program to use these parameters to provide the generalized access method.

### Example 1: Global Open and Push

The simplest method for handling record insertion is to locate the point of insertion in linear address space and to push all the records behind it back the amount of space required to store the new record.

The difficulties with this simple procedure are that (a) it invalidates any physical address pointers pointing to the moved records, (b) it requires a rewrite of all the moved records endangering data integrity, and, perhaps most importantly, (c) it takes a *long* time.

For example, a record insertion using this procedure for a two hundred character record, 100,000 record file stored on an IBM 3330 would require an average minimum move time of about thirty seconds. During this minimum time, no other transactions could be addressed to the file. Clearly this simple procedure would not be useful in a real time system.

### Example 2: Local Open and Push - Embedded Control Field

One way to overcome the gross penalties of Example 1 is to put a bound on the record ripple process. In IBM's Indexed Sequential Access Method, this bound is the end of a prime track; in IBM's VSAM, it is the end of a control interval or control area.

In DIAM II, this bound is realized by defining partitions of the Address Space called *Frames*. These Frames are a generalization of the programming properties of blocks, tracks, cylinders, packs, etc. (On Page 10 under Frame Definition, we present a list of parameters by which the user can specify the size, space handling and overflow handling properties of types of frames. The reader may wish to refer to this list as he follows the next few examples.)

Overflow Procedure Rules

In Example 2 (Figure 3a), a FRAME OVERFLOW Control Field can be defined for each Frame. The purpose of this control field is to provide a means for constructing chains of Frames to contain overflow records. There are two methods to handle the overflowing records: (a) push them one by one into the overflow frames or (b) split the records in the overflowing frame and place half of them in the new frame. The OVERFLOW PROCEDURE parameter (either PUSH RECORDS or SPLIT RECORDS) indicates the user's choice.

There are two ways of terminating the collection of records for a frame

(a) pointing to the last record

(b) placing an FRAME END MARK in the last record.

The first requires a LAST RECORD Control Field for the frame and the second requires the user to define an FRAME END MARK for either the NEXT RECORD POINTER or the RECORD DELETE FIELD.

Another required function is the ability to reserve space at load time. This will be accomplished by allowing prime and overflow space in the composition of each Frame. (designated by either PR or OV in the FRAME COMPOSITION parameters).

In using Example 2 for record insertion, the system never has to ripple records out of more than one original prime Frame.

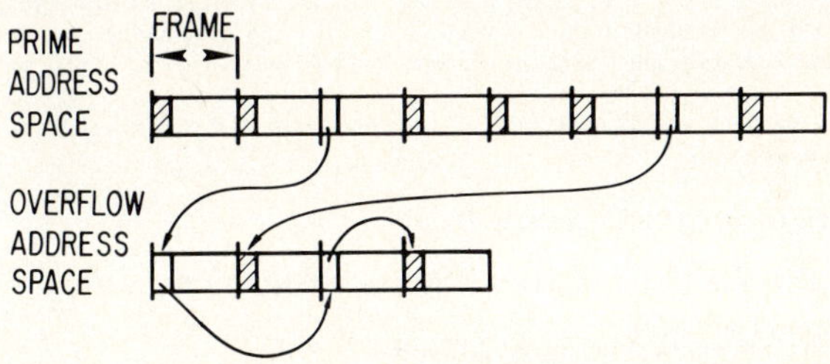


Figure 3a Example 2: Frames and Control Fields on an Address Space

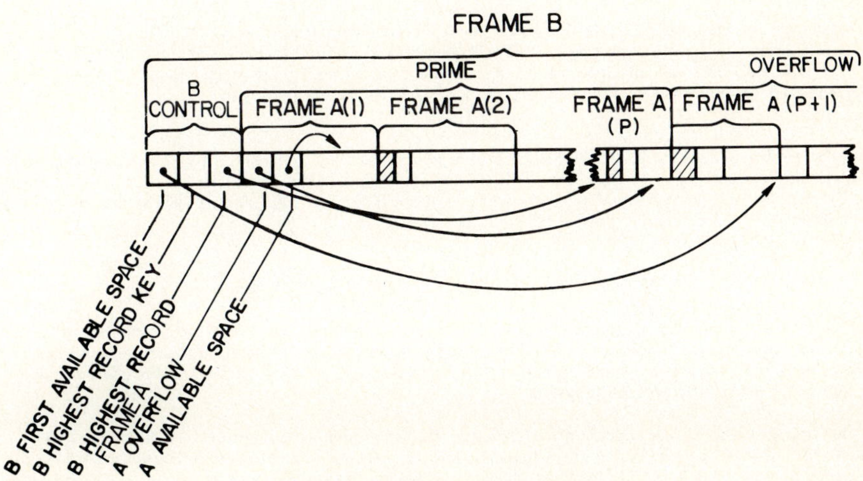


Figure 3b Example 4: A Frame Hierarchy

Example 3: Efficient "Available Space Control" - "Add Onto End" Properties

The location of (a) the first *available space* to insert a record and (b) the *last record* within a particular collection (with the highest (or lowest) key if the records are sorted) are processes that can be accomplished by scanning the address space.

To eliminate scan time, many systems maintain (a) a pointer to the first *available space* (b) a control field containing the value of the *highest (lowest) key* and (c) a control field pointing to the *last record.*

This now gives us four possible control fields to define for a Frame.

(a) FRAME OVERFLOW
(b) AVAILABLE SPACE
(c) HIGHEST (LOWEST) KEY
(d) LAST RECORD

In some cases, the AVAILABLE SPACE Pointer and the Pointer to the back of the LAST RECORD may have the same value. In these cases, one control field will serve both purposes.

Example 4: Hierarchies of Frames

Up to this point we have had only one level and one type of Frame. Most systems have more than one level and type, each with its own specialized, redundant facilities for level specification (For example, IBM VSAM has control intervals and control areas, IBM ISAM has prime frames, overflow frames, and at least two types of index frames.) In DIAM, we avoid this redundancy and gain generality by allowing *recursive* specification of the COMPOSITION of higher level Frames in terms of lower level Frames.

As in Figure 3b, we could have Frame B defined as being composed of Frame A's. Frame B, itself, has embedded control fields which:

(a) contain the HIGHEST KEY in Frame B,

(b) point to the Frame A having the Record with the HIGHEST KEY, and

(c) point to the first Frame A having AVAILABLE SPACE.

Each Frame A could be composed of 10,000 BYTES and have its own set of overflow pointers. In this configuration, we have placed an overflow area in Frame B immediately after the prime area.

The procedure for updating and insertion might have the following appearance. In Figure 3b, A (1) has received an insert and an overflow frame, A (P+1), has been connected to by A (1)'s overflow pointer. A (P+2) is now the first Available Space in B. If a record came in with a key higher than the B HIGHEST RECORD KEY, A (P) would be accessed. If there was space left in this frame, then the new record would be placed there.

If no space were available, the B AVAILABLE SPACE pointer pointing to A (P+2) would be accessed and the record would be placed in A (P+2), the OVERFLOW pointer of A (P) would be set to A (P+2), the B AVAILABLE SPACE pointer would be set to A (P+3), the B HIGHEST KEY control field would be updated, and the B HIGHEST KEY pointer now would point to A (P+2).

## ALLOCATING ADDRESS SPACES TO DEVICES

The definition of a hierarchy of frames is, in essence, a *type* definition because the same definition (like the definition of an access method) can be used to manage record storage for many different address spaces. However, before we can assign a frame definition to an address space, we must specify how the address space is allocated on the physical devices in the system.

A major characteristic of this allocation is that it may be discontinuous with respect to the physical device address space. In the example of "extents" for data sets, the first extent might cover device cylinders 1-7, and the second, device cylinders, 12-14. While there is no reason why address allocation could not be discontinuous to the byte (bit) level, it seems that allocations in terms of blocks (pages), tracks, cylinders, and packs provide a reasonable level of detail.

An example allocation might be ADDRESS SPACE A = (PACK = 7 (CYLINDER = 1,7 (TRACK = 5,9 (BLOCK = 3,6)))) which allocates the address space to pack 7 where the allocation runs through blocks 3 to 6 of track 5 to 9 of cylinders 1 to 7. In this case, the linear address space address = 0 would be the first byte of pack 7, cylinder 1, track 5, block 3.

Normally the highest level frame type of the frame hierarchy would be equated to an *instance* of an ADDRESS SPACE, and the lower level frames would be designed to coincide with the lower level physical subdivisions (tracks and blocks, for example).

## MORE EXAMPLES

Example 5: Fixed Location External Control Fields - A Primary Index Capability

The control fields associated with a particular frame need not be embedded directly in the frame; we can place them in a fixed location in another frame and have an procedural relationship between the location of the control field and the location of its corresponding frame. Figure 4 indicates this configuration.

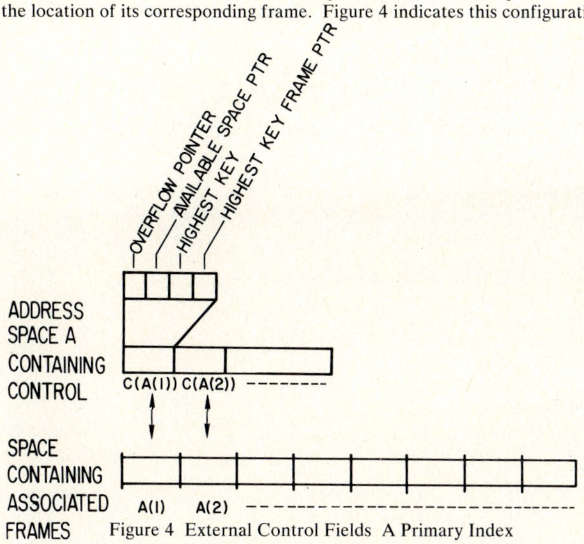


Figure 4 External Control Fields A Primary Index

This example provides a combination of ISAM and VSAM properties.

(a) The control fields rather than the frames themselves can be searched to determine the location of the record sought. (The control field scan is equivalent to an index level scan.)

(b) Overflow is chained out of the prime Frame as in ISAM overflow from the prime track. HIGHEST KEY field need not be updated.

(c) Available space for overflow is obtained by splitting frames and sharing of records (VSAM).

We now have an organization that substantially cuts down on the scanning required to locate a record. (The "index entries" are much smaller than the data frames.) We can, of course, go one step further and, by recursion, define a frame (with its control fields external) on the control field address space to form a "higher level index".

Example 6: Variable Location External Control Fields

In this example as in the case of frame hierachies, we can gain generality and decrease redundancy by noticing that second type of recursion is possible. The combination of external control fields for a frame can be considered as a higher level record with its own primary key. If we now insert this record into the control field address space on the basis of its key, then we get functions equivalent to those of B-trees (21) and close to those of IBM's VSAM.

All we need to more closely approximate VSAM is an intermingling of the control field address space and the data frame address space on the physical device.

With the three building blocks: Address Space, Record, and Frame; five types of control fields and with recursion of these concepts, we have presented a means of defining VSAM for fixed format records. To define a close replica of ISAM, all we need is (a) a HIGHEST KEY field for the highest key pushed out of the frame and (b) record chaining.

This slight modification will be characteristic of the Frame Model. The specification of the functions of what appears to be a completely unique access method will not require the definition of a complete new model. It will only require a slight modification of existing Frame model concepts.

Example 7: Space and Record Handling by Chain

One of the difficulties with the prior examples is that they require movement of records to accommodate insertions. This means that any direct pointers to a record must be updated each time the record moves. Since such updating is a difficult and time consuming process, record movement is essentially incompatible with the use of direct pointers.

One way to overcome this difficulty is to avoid moving records. This can be done by adding a NEXT RECORD Pointer to the RECORD DEFINITION to provide record chaining within a frame. In the record definition, we now have two fields:

(a) A RECORD DELETE control field which indicates whether the record is

 (i) valid information

 (ii) deleted information

 (iii) available space

 (iv) the end of a chain.

(b) A NEXT RECORD Pointer (for pointing to the next record with the possibility of containing an FRAME END MARK for denoting the end of a chain).

In the FRAME DEFINITION, we require a FIRST RECORD control field to point to the first record of the chain.

If we take a single frame, then there are three reasonable combinations of chaining and contiguity for controlling record order and available space.

(a) Records chained to maintain order - available space chained

 In this case, the record chain is searched to determine the chain location for the insert. The first location on the available space chain is used to store the record. The record chain is broken to insert the new record.

(b) Records chained - available space contiguous at end (Deletes marked, but not usable)

 In this case, we assume that all available space is kept at the end of the frame and is pointed to by the AVAILABLE SPACE control field. This results in a situation where noncontiguous deleted space must be marked.

(c) Records chained - available space by scan

 In this case, deletes and available space can have the same marker and delete space can be recovered for insertion of records.

Example 8: Overflow from a Chained Frame

When a chained frame is full, there are a number of possible mechanisms for dealing with the next insert. Some of these, however, involve movement of records (for example, splitting of a frame into two frames). The one that allows retention of fixed record positions is the placement of the new record in some other frame and the connection of the record into the next record frame chain. Whenever record chaining is chosen, it is assumed that the INSERT OVERFLOW PROCEDURE would default to the the placement of the record in the overflow frame.

The INSERT OVERFLOW LOCATION rule will normally include some function of the "instance number" of the original frame which is evaluated to provide the name and "instance number" of the overflow frame. For example, in ISAM cylinder embedded overflow, the overflow area's track addresses are given directly, and its cylinder address is given by the prime track's cylinder address. In ISAM with separate overflow, there is generally only one frame for overflow and all prime tracks point directly to it for available space.

The recognition that the overflow frame for any original frame can be specified in terms of an arithmetic function gives us a general method for clustering records together. We can:

(a) place all overflow records into one large overflow frame, in which case, the records for a particular original frame are likely to be widely separated.

(b) go to the other extreme and have each original frame place its overflow records in its own dedicated set of overflow frames.

(c) have any intermediate situation.

To duplicate ISAM functions, there is one further requirement: there are two HIGHEST KEY control fields, one for the highest key presently in the prime track frame and one for the highest key that has overflowed from the prime track frame. These appear as external control fields which lumped together constitute the "track index".

Example 9: Direct Access Functions - Hash Coding Systems

One way to handle overflow in a hash coding organization is to chain overflow records in a separate overflow area. In this case, we equate one frame type to the prime buckets and a second to the overflow area. This is a straightforward use of the elements we have already defined.

The second method, as exemplified by the scan mode of IBM's BDAM, is to place the overflow records elsewhere in the prime area. The chained submode essentially involves an overflow rule that says: Scan a limited number of frames for a frame that has available space, place the new record into that frame, and make the overflow pointer of the overflowing frame point to the overflow accepting frame. To accommodate this submode, all we need to add is a scan mode for locating available space and a limit parameter on the scan to indicate how many frames are to be scanned before an exception signal is sent to the loader. In the so-called progressive overflow method, we simply ignore the use of pointers.

Example 10: Variable Length Records

We have now specified a mechanism and building blocks for handling fixed format records. We have not yet discussed the variable size, variable format records of the type found in IMS, GIS, MARK IV, the DBTG report, IDS, TDMS, etc. These systems provide an additional crucial level of performance by allowing all information about a particular entity to be kept on the same page.

In our framework, these functions are accommodated by including RECORD CODE, and RECORD SIZE fields in the Record Definition.

Another interesting function is called Record Spanning. That is, allowing a record to span the boundary between two frames. This function would be handled by placing a SPAN or NO SPAN parameter in the OVERFLOW PROCEDURE for the Frame. If the second frame may be directly accessed without decoding the first frame, then it must have a control field that points to the first full record in the frame. Such a control field has already been defined.

## REVIEW OF FRAME SPECIFICATIONS

We can now review the parameters defined for frame building blocks. In one sense, this seems to be a large list. On the other hand, it is quite small in comparison to the list that would be required to cover four or five specialized access methods. The equivalent of a particular access method would be achieved in DIAM by writing a macroinstruction which would give default values to most of the paramenters mentioned below and the small number of remaining parameters would be presented for specification by the user.

```
FRAME NAME = frame name

COMPOSITION = n { frame name 1 {PR | OV} [, m frame name 2 {PR | OV}]...
                  {BYTES | BITS} {PR | OV} }

KEY SORT ORDER = { ASC | DESC | FRONT | BACK }

CREATE OVERFLOW LOCATION = (for each lower level frame type in this
                           frame that is likely to overflow on loading,
                           a procedure that gives the overflow frame's
                           number)

INSERT OVERFLOW LOCATION = { (for each lower level frame type in this
                             frame that is likely to overflow on insertion,
                             a procedure that gives the overflow frame's
                             number)
                             [SCAN n RECORDS] }

INSERT OVERFLOW PROCEDURE = { PUSH RECORDS | SPLIT RECORDS }

AVAILABLE SPACE PROCEDURE = { CONTIGUITY | CHAIN } frame-name-1 [, frame-name-2]...

                            ORIGIN  frame-name-1 (frame-number)

CFLOCATION = { (for each lower level frame type that has fixed position
               external control fields, a procedure for placing the
               control field record)
               INSERT frame-name CONTROL FIELDS IN address-space-name }
```

(for a FRAME NAME control fields may be specified by)

```
CONTROL FIELD NAME = control field name

CFSIZE = n { BYTES | BITS }

CFTYPE = { FRAME POINTER
           AVAILABLE SPACE [LAST RECORD]
           {HIGHEST | LOWEST} KEY {IN FRAME | OUT OF FRAME}
           FIRST RECORD
           LAST RECORD {FRONT | BACK} {IN FRAME | OUT OF FRAME}
           OVERFLOW FRAME
           OVERFLOW RECORD }  LOCATION = { IN FRAME | OUT FRAME | CATALOG }

CFPOINTER FORMAT = (similar to DIAM pointer parameters)
```

(for records within the Frame)

```
     RECORD DELETE FIELD SIZE = n  { BYTES }
                                   { BITS  }

     DELETE FIELD FRAME END MARK = frame end mark

     RECORD CODE SIZE = n  { BYTES }
                           { BITS  }

     NEXT RECORD POINTER FORMAT = (similar to DIAM pointer parameters)

     NEXT RECORD FRAME END MARK = frame end code
```

(for each record type)

```
     RECORD CODE code 1 = record type name 1

     RECORD KEY code 1 = field name 1 [, field name 2] ...

     RECORD SIZE code 1 = { SIZE = field size value, UNITS = { BYTES } }
                          {                                 { BITS  } }
                          { VALUE = fixed size value,                 }
                          {                                           }
                          {         COUNTUNITS =  { BYTES }           }
                          {                       { BITS  }           }
```

## COMMENTS ON FRAME DEFINITION

### COMPOSITION

At the lowest level (usually corresponding to the physical device page), the frame composition is expressed in terms of bytes or bits assigned to prime or overflow space. The composition of higher frame levels is expressed in terms of lower level frames. In this definition we have given only a simple possible specification. In an actual system, it would be useful to have the capability of using parentheses as we have in the case of address space allocation to more easily deal with repeating configurations.

### KEY SORT ORDER

FRONT and BACK imply chronological placement of the record either first or last in the frame. In either case the key need not be defined. The default for KEY SORT ORDER should probably be ASC.

### OVERFLOW LOCATION

The procedure could be as simple as supplying the name and number of a single frame instance. Among other things, it could also require division of this frame's instance number to obtain an integer instance number for the overflow frame.

The rules and procedures for overflow from a particular Frame Name will always be placed in the next higher level Frame. In this fashion, we will be able to define particular Frame Types at one level and then use then in two different frames at a higher level.

For example, we might define a Frame Type A at the low level (for example, corresponding to a prime track in ISAM) and want to use it in two different types of Frames at a higher level, say Frame Type B and Frame Type C. In Frame Type B, we would want to overflow to a Frame Type D (for example, cylinder overflow). In Frame Type C, we would want it to overflow to a Frame Type E (separate overflow). In the case, we have mentioned the definition of Frame Type A could be used for both higher level frames.

### OVERFLOW PROCEDURE

This would only be required when contiguity is used for space control. When chains are used to connect records, the assumption would be that the new record would be placed in the overflow area if no space existed for it in the prime frame.

AVAILABLE SPACE PROCEDURE

The AVAILABLE SPACE PROCEDURE will handle available space by either contiguity or chains. In either case, when a frame is removed from the front of available space the pointer will move to the next frame. It will march one by one through the frame types listed in address space order. It will start at the frame given by origin. Both create and insert overflow may use the available space pointer.

CFLOCATION

The default on this would be to place any control fields defined into the front of the frame being defined. If "INSERT address space name" is used then the control fields will be treated as a record and inserted into the designated address space.

CFTYPE

The FRAME POINTER is used when the control fields are stored externally in a movable position as in VSAM and B-Trees. It contains the address space location of its Frame. In the case of the AVAILABLE SPACE type, it is possible that the same pointer would also point to the back of the LAST RECORD. The use of LAST RECORD would indicate this dual purpose possibility. OVERFLOW FRAME would indicate that the control field points to a frame while OVERFLOW RECORD would indicate it points to a particular record in a frame.

CFPOINTER FORMAT

The DIAM pointer format includes the possibility for specifying address spaces and displacements of various sorts within the address spaces. If the pointer always points to the same address space then this information can be factored into the frame description.

RECORD CODE SIZE

Record codes are required only when more than one type of record is to be placed in the frame.

NEXT RECORD POINTER

NEXT RECORD POINTER implies that the records are to be connected by a chain. It also implies that the INSERT OVERFLOW PROCEDURE will place overflowing records directly into the overflow space and connect them into the record chain at the appropriate position. If it does not exist then contiguity is implied.

We have now given the specifications for the frames; we will now indicate how a program could read these descriptions and manage record placement.

## FRAME PARAMETER EXAMPLES

A SEQUENTIAL FILE

```
FRAME NAME = SEQFILE

    COMPOSITION =  500 SEQBLOCK PR

    KEY SORT ORDER = ASC

    CREATE OVERFLOW LOCATION = FRAME TYPE = SEQBLOCK
                                 OVERFLOW = AVAILABLE SPACE POINTER

    AVAILABLE SPACE PROCEDURE = CONTIGUITY SEQBLOCK
                                ORIGIN SEQBLOCK (0)

    CFTYPE = AVAILABLE SPACE  LOCATION = CATALOG

    RECORD KEY = EMP-NO

    RECORD SIZE = VALUE = 200 COUNTUNITS = BYTES.
```

```
FRAME NAME = SEQBLOCK

    COMPOSITION = 1000 BYTES
```

This is a sequential file of Employee records with 200 byte records, and 500 SEQBLOCK's of 1000 bytes each.

Two Level B-Tree

For the data records, we define a DATABLK frame type which is contained in a higher frame, DATAFILE.

```
FRAME NAME = DATAFILE

    COMPOSITION = 500 DATABLK

    KEY SORT ORDER = ASC

    CREATE OVERFLOW LOCATION = FRAME TYPE = DATABLK
                               OVERFLOW = AVAILABLE SPACE POINTER

    INSERT OVERFLOW LOCATION = FRAME TYPE = DATABLK
                               OVERFLOW = AVAILABLE SPACE POINTER

    INSERT OVERFLOW PROCEDURE = SPLIT RECORDS

    AVAILABLE SPACE PROCEDURE = CONTIGUITY DATABLK
                               ORIGIN = DATABLK (0)

    CFLOCATION = INSERT DATABLK CONTROL FIELDS IN INDEX1SPACE

    RECORD KEY = DEPT-NO

    RECORD SIZE = VALUE = 100 COUNTUNITS = BYTES

FRAME NAME = DATABLK

    COMPOSITION = 1000 BYTES PR

    CONTROL FIELD NAME = DATAHK
    CFSIZE = 3 BYTES
    CFTYPE = HIGHEST KEY IN FRAME  LOCATION OUT FRAME
    CFPOINTER FORMAT = see BEU pointer format

    CONTROL FIELD NAME = DATAFPTR
    CFSIZE = 6 BYTES
    CFTYPE = FRAME POINTER  LOCATION = OUT FRAME
    CFPOINTER FORMAT = see BEU pointer
```

Next, we wish to define the first level index in terms of INDEX1 and INDEXBLK frames.

```
FRAME NAME = INDEX1

    COMPOSITION = 5 INDEXBLK PR

    KEY SORT ORDER = ASC

    CREATE OVERFLOW LOCATION = FRAME TYPE = INDEXBLK
                               OVERFLOW = AVAILABLE SPACE POINTER

    INSERT OVERFLOW LOCATION = FRAME TYPE = INDEXBLK
                               OVERFLOW = AVAILABLE SPACE POINTER
```

```
    INSERT OVERFLOW PROCEDURE = SPLIT RECORDS

    AVAILABLE SPACE PROCEDURE = CONTIGUITY INDEXBLK
                                ORIGIN = INDEXBLK (0)

    CFLOCATION = INSERT INDEXBLK CONTROL FIELDS IN INDEX2SPACE

    RECORD KEY = DATAHK

    RECORD SIZE = VALUE = 9 COUNTUNITS = BYTES

FRAME NAME = INDEXBLK

    COMPOSITION = 1000 BYTES PR

    CONTROL FIELD NAME = INDEX1HK
    CFSIZE = 3 BYTES
    CFTYPE = HIGHEST KEY IN FRAME  LOCATION = OUT FRAME
    CFPOINTER FORMAT = see BEU format

    CONTROL FIELD NAME = INDEX1FPTR
    CFSIZE = 6 BYTES
    CFTYPE = FRAME POINTER LOCATION = OUT FRAME
    CFPOINTER FORMAT = see BEU format
```

And finally, we need one block to contain the second level index.

```
FRAME NAME = INDEX2

    COMPOSITION = 100 BYTES PR

    KEY SORT ORDER = ASC

    RECORD KEY = INDEX1HK

    RECORD SIZE = VALUE = 9 COUNTUNITS = BYTES
```

## MECHANISM TO SUPPORT RECORD PLACEMENT

Associated with each record type to be placed will be an Address Space Name. This will lead to a set of frame definitions for the address space. (For example, the definitions might be for an ISAM type specification.) In the simple case of Record Order either FRONT or BACK, the system would not require a key; it would place the record either at the front or back of the frame.

If the record has a key, then the system will:

Step 1:

Check a system mode bit for the initial frame to determine whether create overflow rules are to be used. If they are then it will go to step 2, if not it will go to step 3.

Step 2: Create Mode

If there is a HIGHEST (LOWEST) KEY for this frame, test the new record's key against it.

If the new record key is high (or low) use the LAST RECORD pointer to locate the former highest key record and place the new record after it using first available space or overflow rules. Update AVAILABLE SPACE pointer, HIGHEST KEY and LAST RECORD pointer and return.

If the new record key is Low (or High) use Insert Mode (Step 3).

Step 3: Insert Mode

If there are lower level frames composing this frame, determine whether they have any HIGH KEY control field (external or embedded). If they have external fields, then look to see if the frames to which the external fields are assigned have their own external HIGH KEY control field. Follow this recursion to the highest level, then compare the new record key with the HIGHEST KEY fields; back down the "index levels" to determine the particular lowest level frame instance which contains the appropriate location for the new record.

Whenever the HIGHEST KEY control field is embedded, use a scan of the embedded fields to locate the appropriate frame instance. In there are no HIGHEST KEY control fields, then simply scan the record instances themselves to find the insert point.

This process gives us the record before and the record behind the new record. (Non-unique keys require a slight extension of the definition of the definition of "before" and "behind".) We now consult the AVAILABLE SPACE rules to determine how to insert the record.

(a) If chaining is used to control record order, then select the first available space, place the record into it, and insert the record into the record chain. Update available space indicators.

If no available space exists in this frame, use overflow rules to find available space, place the record into the available space, and chain into the record chain. Update available space and overflow indicators.

(b) If contiguity is used, then use open and push to make room for the new record. If a record is pushed out of the frame, then use the overflow rule to find a place for it. In this case the HIGHEST KEY control field may have to be updated. In any case, the AVAILABLE SPACE indicators are updated.

## SUMMARY

In this paper, we have defined three building blocks with recursion for constructing a very general set of record storage mechanisms. These building blocks are supported by a relatively simple interpretive mechanism for searching and maintaining the record storage organization.

This work is compatible with the higher levels of the DIAM system and constitutes a detailed, parameterized description of its lowest level, the Physical Device Level.

## ACKNOWLEDGEMENT

We would like to thank our referee for a number of suggestions including the suggestion that examples of the use of FRAME parameter be included. Construction of these examples has helped us to refine the parameter list.

*References*

(1) S. E. Madnick, J. W. Alsop: A modular approach to file system design. SJCC, 1969, 1-13.

(2) H. S. Meltzer: Data base concepts and architecture for data base systems, IBM Report to SHARE Information Systems Research Project (August 20, 1969).

(3) M. E. Senko, E. B. Altman, M. M. Astrahan, and P. L. Fehder: Data structures and accessing in data base systems. IBM Systems J. 1973, 12, 30-93.

(4) G. H. Mealy: Another look at data, FJCC 1967, pp. 525-534.

(5) C. W. Bachman: Trends in database management-1975. Proceedings of the 1975 National Computer Conference, pp 569-576 (AFIPS Press, Montvale, New Jersey, 1975).

SPARC interim report, American National Standards Institute Document No. 7514TS01 (ANSI, Washington, D. C., Feb. 8,1975).

(6) R. E. Levien and M. E. Maron: A computer system for inference execution and data retrieval. Comm ACM, 1967, 10, 715-721.

(7) B. Langefors: Information systems. Information Processing 74, 937-945 (North-Holland, Amsterdam, 1974).

(8) B. Sundgren: An Infological Approach to Data Bases. (Urval nr 7) (National Central Bureau of Statistics, Stockholm, Sweden, 1973).

(9) J. R. Abrial: Data Semantics. IFIP-TC-2 Working Conference on "Data Base Management Systems", Cargese, Corsica (North Holland, Amsterdam).

(10) M. E. Senko: The DDL in the context of a multilevel structured description: DIAM II with FORAL, Data Base Description, B.C.M. Douque and G.M. Nijssen (eds.). pp. 239-240 (North Holland Publishing Co., Amsterdam, 1975).

(11) M. E. Senko: Specification of stored data structures and desired output results in DIAM II with FORAL, Proc. ACM Conference on Very Large Data Bases (ACM, New York, 1975).

(12) M. E. Senko: DIAM as a detailed example of the ANSI SPARC architecture, Proceedings of the IFIP TC-2 Working Conference on Modelling in Data Base Management Systems, Freudenstadt, Germany, January 5-9, 1976 (North-Holland, Amsterdam).

(13) G. K. Manacher: On the feasibility of implementing a large relational data base with optimal performance on a mini-computer, Proceedings of the International Conference on Very Large Data Bases 175-201 (ACM, New York, 1975).

(14) H. A. Schmid and P. A. Bernstein: A multi-level architecture for relational data base systems, Proceedings of the International Conference on Very Large Data Bases, 202-226 (ACM, New York, 1975).

(15) D. Tsichritzis: Features of a conceptual schema, Proceedings of the International Conference on Very Large Data Bases, 532-534 (ACM, New York, 1975).

(16) D. Hsiao and F. Harary: A formal system for information retrieval from files, ACM Comm. 13, No. 2, 67-73 (February, 1970).

(17) D. P. Smith: An approach to data description and conversion, Moore School Report No. 72-20 (University of Pennsylvannia, 1971).

(18) R. W. Taylor and E. H. Sibley: A data definition and mapping language, ACM Comm. 16, 750-759 (December, 1973).

(19) L. S. Schneider: A relational view of the data independent accessing model, Proc. 1976 SIGMOD International Conference on Management of Data, Washington, D. C., 75-90 (ACM, New York, 1976).

(20) M. E. Senko and E. B. Altman: DIAM Note 1: A framework mode for implementing a record-storing facility, RJ 1365 (IBM Research, Yorktown Heights, New York, 1972).

(21) R. Bayer and E. McCreight: Organization and maintenance of large ordered indexes, Acta Informatica 1, 173-189 (1972).

*Systems for Large Data Bases, P.C. Lockemann and E.J. Neuhold, (eds.)*
*North-Holland Publishing Company, 1976*

# RELATIONS TRANSFORMATION AND A REDUNDANCY IN RELATIONAL DATA BASE

E. L. Lozinskii
Department of Computer Science
The Hebrew University
Jerusalem, Israel.

This paper considers some transformation and replacement of relations in a relational data base, called association and dissociation, which are intended to decrease the time of jobs processing and files updating, although it is accompanied by an increase of information redundancy. Some examples are examined. It is shown that in a considerable number of practical cases association and dissociation are effective means of processing time reduction and data base adaptation.

The efficiency of a relational data base depends on its set of relations [1-6,9,10]. Since a given set of jobs to be solved by a system does not determine unambiguously the set of required relations, it is necessary to form the set of relations, so that certain performance criteria are satisfied.

Suppose that a data base contains a set of relations $\{R_i\}$, presented in the third normal form, with the relation $R_i$ containing a set of domains $\{D_{ij}\}$. The data base is used by a set of jobs $\{J_j\}_{j=1}^{m}$, and $p_j$ is the frequency of processing of the job $J_j$. Let $R_1,R_2,\ldots,R_r$ be joinable relations [1], and $R_s$ (where $s$ is a list of indices $1,2,\ldots,r$) is a join of relations $R_1,R_2,\ldots,R_r$ in the sense that each of this relations can be derived as a certain projection of $R_s$: $R_i = \pi_i(R_s)$. It is evident that by replacing in the data base the relations $R_1,R_2,\ldots,R_r$ by the relation $R_s$, we obtain a new version of the set of relations $\{R_i\}$, that is still sufficient for processing of jobs $J_j$. Such replacement of joinable relations by their join will be called an <u>association</u> of relations in a data base (fig. 1). Let $R_i^{(1)},R_i^{(2)},\ldots,R_i^{(\ell)}$ be projections of a relation $R_i$, that form a full set of projections of $R_i$ in the sense that $R_i$ can be derived as a certain join of $R_i^{(1)},R_i^{(2)},\ldots,R_i^{(\ell)}$. By replacing in the data base the relation $R_i$ by the relations $R_i^{(1)},R_i^{(2)},\ldots,R_i^{(\ell)}$ we obtain a new relations set $\{R_i\}$ that is still sufficient for processing of jobs $\{J_j\}$. Such replacement of a relation by its full set of projections will be called a dissociation of relations in a data base (fig.1). It should be noted, that association can cause a transition of relations from the third normal form to the second normal form (e.g. $R_1(\underline{D_1},D_2)$, $R_2(\underline{D_2},D_3)$, $R_s(\underline{D_1},D_2,D_3)$, the primary key is underlined) or to the first normal form (e.g. $R_1(\underline{D_1,D_2},D_3)$, $R_2(\underline{D_2},D_4)$, $R_s(\underline{D_1,D_2},D_3,D_4)$).

Our aim is to determine the conditions of usefulness of association and dissociation of relations according to the following data base performance criterion: the total processing time of jobs processing and relations updating. We shall use the following notation: $N_i$ is the number of tuples in $R_i$; $n_i^j$ is the number of tuples of $R_i$ processed by the job $J_j$; $t_i$ is the scanning time of $R_i$; $v_i$ is the size of $R_i$; $K_i = t_i/t_s = v_i/v_s$; $q_i$ is the frequency of updating of $R_i$; $n_i^u$ is the number of tuples processed when updating $R_i$; $\varepsilon < 1$ is the coefficient which takes into account an improvement of performance achieved by an appropriate job ordering.

The total processing time of relations $R_1,R_2,\ldots,R_r$ during a time unit of a system operation:

$$T_1 = \sum_{i=1}^{r} \frac{t_i}{N_i} (q_i n_i^u + \varepsilon \sum_{j=1}^{m} p_j n_i^j)$$

$$= \sum_{i=1}^{r} t_i (q_i \alpha_i^u + \varepsilon \sum_{j=1}^{m} p_j \alpha_i^j), \quad \text{where} \quad \alpha_i^j = \frac{n_i^j}{N_i}.$$

The total processing time of their join $R_s$:

$$T_2 = t_s (q_s \alpha_s^u + \varepsilon \sum_{j=1}^{m} p_j \alpha_s^j).$$

Then the condition of useful association is:

$$T_2 < T_1$$

$$\varepsilon \sum_{j=1}^{m} p_j (\alpha_s^j - \sum_{i=1}^{r} K_i \alpha_i^j) < \sum_{i=1}^{r} K_i q_i \alpha_i^u - q_s \alpha_s^u \qquad (1)$$

The condition of useful dissociation:

$$T_1 < T_2 \qquad (2)$$

So the third normal form may be considered as an intermediate point for further constructing of relations by means of association and dissociation in order to improve performance by taking into account not only a data structure but also the parameters of jobs and updating flow (fig. 2).

As an illustration we shall examine a simplest practical example of two joinable relations $R_1$ and $R_2$, and their join $R_s$. Let A be a set of jobs which use $R_1$ and don't use $R_2$, B is a set of jobs which use $R_2$ and don't use $R_1$, C is a set of jobs which use $R_s$ (or both of $R_1$ and $R_2$). Let us denote by $n_y^{(x)}$ the expected number of tuples of $R_y$ processed by a job $J \in x$:

$$n_y^{(x)} = \frac{\sum_{J_i \in x} p_i n_y^i}{\sum_{J_i \in x} p_i} ; \quad \alpha_y^{(x)} = \frac{n_y^{(x)}}{N_y} \quad \text{for } y=1,2,s; \; x = A,B,C$$

The condition (1) will assume the form:

$$\varepsilon((\alpha_s^{(A)} - K_1\alpha_1^{(A)}) \sum_{J_i \in A} p_i + (\alpha_s^{(B)} - K_2\,\alpha_2^{(B)}) \sum_{J_i \in B} p_i \tag{3}$$

$$+ (\alpha_s^{(C)} - K_1\,\alpha_1^{(C)} - K_2\,\alpha_2^{(C)}) \sum_{J_i \in C} p_i) < K_1 q_1 \alpha_1^u + K_2 q_2 \alpha_2^u - q_s \alpha_s^u$$

In order to evaluate $\alpha_s^{(A)}$ and $\alpha_s^{(B)}$ let us note that if a job $J_j \in A$ is referred to $R_s$, there are two possibilities:

a) to process directly the relation $R_s$ which requires a time $\alpha_1^{(A)} t_s$,

b) to obtain $R_1$ as a projection of $R_s$ (during one scan of $R_s$) and then to process $R_1$, which requires a time $t_s + \alpha_1^{(A)} t_1$.

The choice of either possibility is determined by the sign of the difference $\alpha_1^{(A)} t_s - (t_s + \alpha_1^{(A)} t_1) = t_s(\alpha_1^{(A)}(1-K_1)-1)$. Hence,

$$\alpha_s^{(A)} = \begin{cases} 1 + K_1\,\alpha_1^{(A)} & \text{for } K_1 < 1 - 1/\alpha_1^{(A)} \\ \alpha_1^{(A)} & \text{for } K_1 \geq 1 - 1/\alpha_1^{(A)} \end{cases} \tag{4}$$

The number of tuples $n_i^j$ processed by $J_j$ consists of the number of tuples required by the job and the number of tuples accessed during sorting if $J_j$ changes the order of the tuples of $R_i$.

Considering that the expected number of tuples of $R_i$ required by $J_j$ is $0.5\ N_i$ (it corresponds both to normal and to uniform distribution of $n_i^j$), and that practically sorting accounts for about 20% of data processing jobs requiring on the average about five scans of a file to be sorted [7,8], we derive: $\alpha_1^{(A)} = \alpha_2^{(B)} = \alpha_s^{(C)} = 1.5$, $\alpha_1^{(C)} = \alpha_2^{(C)} = 2.0$. By assuming that all the values of $K_1 (0 < K_1 < 1)$ are equiprobable, we obtain from (4) $\alpha_s^{(A)} = \alpha_s^{(B)} = 1.13$ (if the values of $K_1$ are distributed according to the normal law, then $\alpha_s^{(A)} = \alpha_s^{(B)} = 1.18$). Let us denote $K = (K_1 + K_2)/2$,

$$Q = (q_1\alpha_1^u + q_2\,\alpha_2^u)/(\sum_{J_i\in A} p_i + \sum_{J_i\in B} p_i + \sum_{J_i\in C} p_i),$$

$$G_x = \sum_{J_i\in x} p_i \,/\, (\sum_{J_i\in A} p_i + \sum_{J_i\in B} p_i + \sum_{J_i\in C} p_i) \quad \text{for } x = A,B,C.$$

Then considering that the amount of updating of a relation is proportional to the size of this relation, we derive, from (3) the following condition:

$$\begin{aligned} &\varepsilon(\alpha_s^{(A)}(1 - G_C) + \alpha_1^{(A)}\ (G_C - K_1G_A - K_2G_B) - \\ &2\,\alpha_1^{(C)}\ K\,G_C) < Q(2K - (1 + 2K_1K_2)/2K) \end{aligned} \tag{5}$$

By assuming for simplicity that $\varepsilon = 1$, $G_A \approx G_B$, $G_C = G$ we obtain from (5) the following approximate condition which is nevertheless sufficient for illustrating the result:

$$G(0.185\text{-}1.25K) - 0.75K + 0.565 < Q(K\text{-}0.38/K) \tag{6}$$

According to our consideration each pair of relations is characterized by a triplet $(K,Q,G)$ and can be represented as a point of a three-dimensional space. Fig.3 gives the plot of the function

$$G(0.185\text{-}1.25K) - 0.75K + 0.565 - Q(K - 0.38/K) = 0 \tag{7}$$

Points of the space "above the surface" have coordinates satisfying (6) and consequently correspond to useful association of relations. In order to evaluate the expediency of association of relations let us examine the probability $P_a$ of useful association in the sense of (1) of two joinable relations of a data base. Suppose that for the relations of the data base under consideration hold $K' \leq K \leq K''$, $G' \leq G \leq G''$, $Q' \leq Q \leq Q''$. Then assuming that values of $K,G,Q$ are uniformly distributed in the corresponding intervals, we determine:

$$P_a = 1 - \frac{1}{(K''-K')(G''-G')(Q''-Q')} \iint\limits_{\substack{G' \leq G \leq G'' \\ Q' \leq Q \leq Q''}} K^* \, dG \, dQ, \tag{8}$$

where $K,G,Q$ satisfy the equation (7) and

$$K^* = \begin{cases} 0 & \text{for } K < K' \\ K-K' & \text{for } K' \leq K \leq K'' \\ K''-K' & \text{for } K > K'' \end{cases}$$

By analogy with (8) we evaluate also the probability $P_d$ of useful dissociation of an arbitrary relation in the sense of (2), considering $K > 0.5$. Indeed, if $R_1$ and $R_2$ constitute a full set of projections of $R_3$, have the same primary key, and contain all the domains of $R_3$, then $v_1 + v_2 > v_3$.

Table 1 contains the values of $P_a$ and $P_d$ for several concrete examples:

1) general case,
2) static relation with low frequency of updating $Q$,
3) dynamic relation with a high frequency of updating $Q$,
4) "joint" relations with a high frequency of joint processing $G$,
5) "separate" relations with a low frequency of joint processing $G$,
6) reference relations (which are used only for checking and duplication of working relations) with a very low frequency of joint processing and relatively high frequency of updating.

Table 1. The probability of useful association and dissociation.

| Characteristic of relations | Parameters | $P_a$ $0 < K < 1$ | $P_d$ $0.5 < K < 1$ |
|---|---|---|---|
| General case | $0 < G < 1$<br>$0 < Q < 1$ | 0.42 | 0.14 |
| Static | $0 < G < 1$<br>$0 < Q < 0.1$ | 0.48 | 0.11 |
| Dynamic | $0 < G < 1$<br>$1 < Q < 10$ | 0.39 | 0.22 |
| Joint | $0.5 < G < 1$<br>$0 < Q < 1$ | 0.54 | 0.02 |
| Separate | $0 < G < 0.5$<br>$0 < Q < 1$ | 0.30 | 0.42 |
| Reference | $G \approx 0$<br>$0 < Q < 10$ | 0.28 | 0.44 |

An analysis of the condition (1),(2) and of the graphs leads to the following conclusions:

1) In a considerable number of practical cases the association and dissociation of relations in a data base are effective methods of reduction of a total processing time of jobs processing and relations updating, although it causes a certain increase of an information redundancy and a transition of some relations from the third normal form to the second or first normal form;

2) The association is most useful for relations that are processed jointly and for static relations; the dissociation is most useful for reference relations and for relations that are processed separately;

3) Since a set of jobs, their frequency, and frequency of updating change during a system operation, the association and dissociation of relations can be used as means of a data base adaptation during the system evolution.

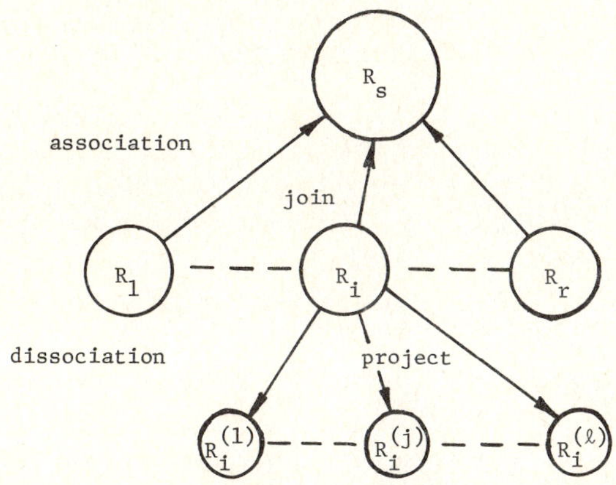


Fig. 1. Association and dissociation of relations.

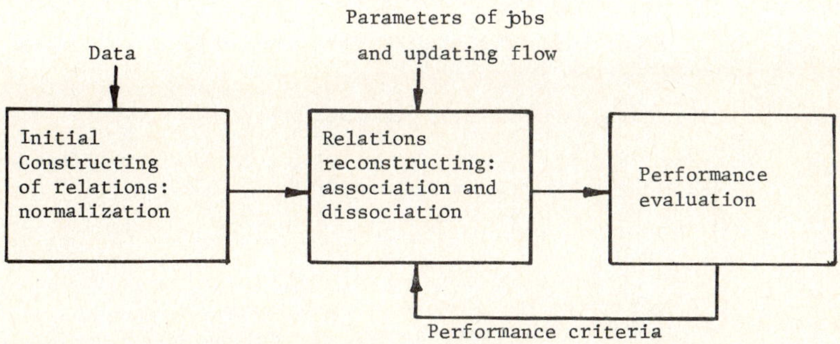


Fig. 2. Adaptive reconstructing of relations.

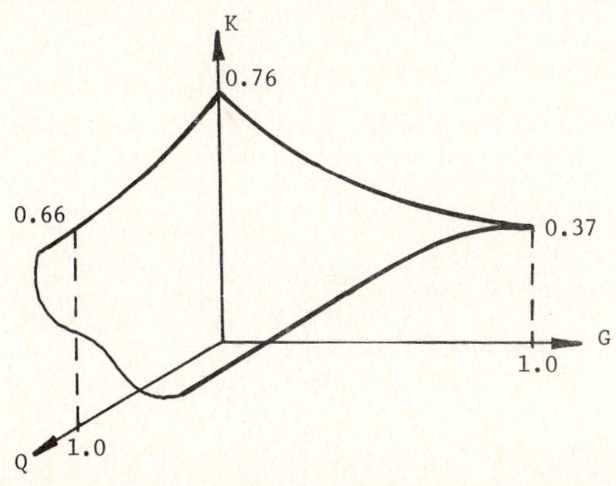


Fig. 3. The space of association/dissociation.

## References

1. Codd, E.F. (1970). A Relational Model of Data for Large Shared Data Banks; CACM, 13, No.6, 377-387.

2. Codd, E.F. (1972). Further Normalization of the Data Base Relational Model; in "Data Base Systems", Courant Computer Science Symposia Series, 6, 33-64.

3. Codd, E.F. (1974). Recent Investigations in Relational Data Base Systems; Proc. IFIP Congress (North-Holland, Amsterdam).

4. Date, C.J., and Codd, E.F. (1974). The Relational and Network Approaches; IBM Report RJ 1401.

5. Date, C.J. (1975). An Introduction to Database Systems (Addison-Wesley).

6. Date, C.J. (1976). Relational Data Base Concepts; Datamation, 22, No.4, 50-53.

7. Knuth, D.E. (1973). The Art of Computer Programming, v.3 (Addison-Wesley).

8. Lozinskii, L.S. (1968). An Analysis of External Merge Sorting Techniques; Cybernetics, 4, No.1, 21-28.

9. Martin, J. (1975). Computer Data-Base Organization (Prentice-Hall).

10. Senko, M.E. (1975). Information Systems: Records, Relations, Sets, Entities, and Things; Information Systems, 1, No.1, 3-14.

*Systems for Large Data Bases, P.C. Lockemann and E.J. Neuhold, (eds.)*
*North-Holland Publishing Company, 1976*

# HIGH PERFORMANCE HARDWARE FOR DATABASE SYSTEMS

D.R. McGregor, R.G. Thomson, W.N. Dawson
Department of Computer Science
University of Strathclyde
Glasgow, Scotland.

The work is founded on a comprehensive database model which provides various user languages and supports different "views" of the data. The low-level database structure is based on the n-ary relational model.

A special-purpose processor is described which can directly perform the relational primitive operations.

Novel algorithms for these operations are outlined.

## 1. INTRODUCTION

Some years ago Codd (1970, 1972) published an important series of papers introducing the concepts of relational databases. He postulated an abstract database in which information is held as a set of relations each consisting of a set of tuples. To specify data manipulation operations Codd defined a set of relational operators - Restriction, Projection, Join, etc., by which specific subsets of tuples can be selected, subsets of attributes can be extracted or information in one or more relations can be correlated.

There have been two different and general reactions to Codd's proposals. First it is widely agreed that, in principle, the relational model is a major advance in the theory of databases. But secondly, as far as implementation is concerned considerable doubt has been expressed about the practicality of the ideas.

Another difficulty is that databases are required to support database languages founded on concepts other than the n-ary relational one proposed by Codd. Our own work is based on the conceptual model given in Figure 1.

Various database languages can be employed by the user to specify the data manipulations he requires in terms of his own data sub-model (or "view" of the data). Statements in the user language are then translated into a common interface language (though still expressed in terms of the user's own view). The Intermediate level of the model using catalogued information remaps the operations in terms of the global data model, i.e. the user's command is now expressed in terms of operations on information actually stored within the database. Considerable optimisation of the commands is then possible. Some manipulations may be found to be unnecessary in that they cancel each other out. It is also usually possible to re-arrange the order of the instructions so that the amount of work needed to carry them out is greatly reduced. At the lowest level of the model we have an "Abstract Database Machine", which executes strings of commands produced by the higher levels.

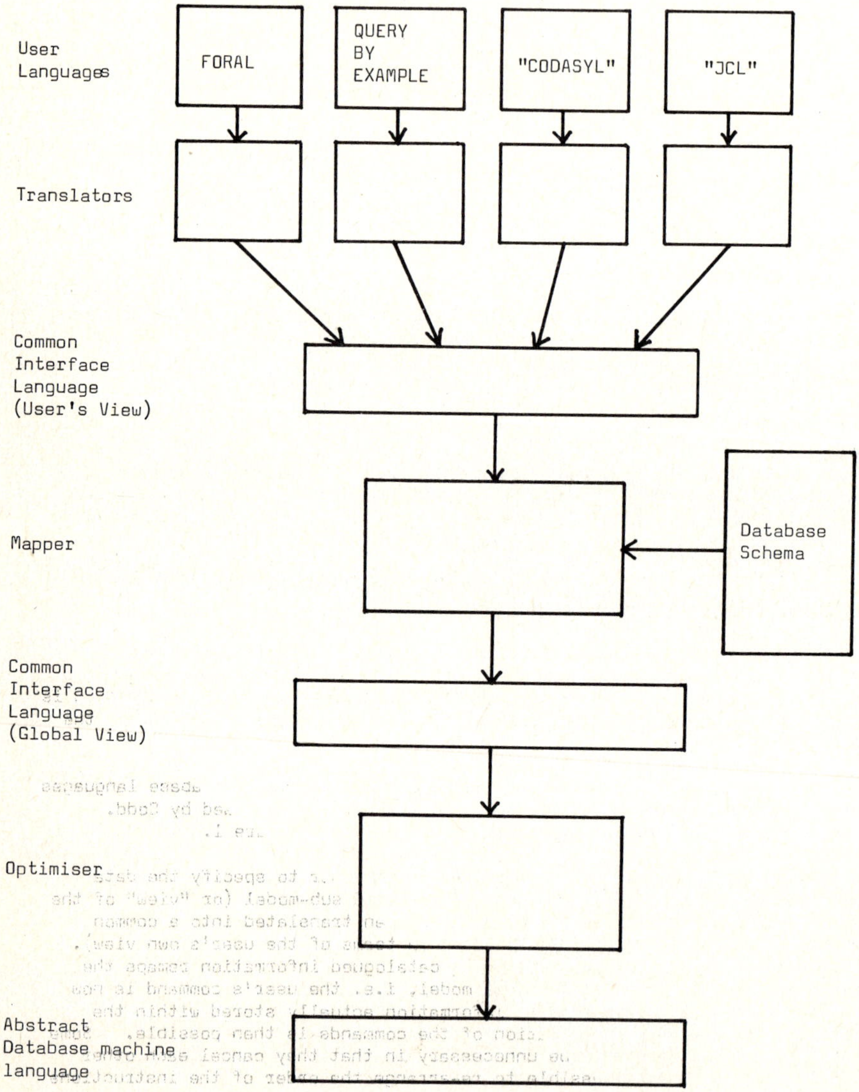


Fig. 1 Database Architecture

The aim of our research is to realise this conceptual model in a practical form. We see the "Abstract Database Machine" essentially as a "Codd machine". There is, however, no accepted way of implementing a general relational database except at the cost of considerable inefficiency (although the PRTV system (Todd, 1975) is fairly successful in several respects). Existing practical (non-relational) databases allow user programs to find their own way about the data, thus limiting the "data structure independence" of the programs, while many proposed relational databases depend on previously prepared navigational information such as directories or pointers. In the latter case possible paths through the data tend to be restricted to those already signposted thus destroying the generality which is an important feature of the relational ideas. As it seems likely, however, that a general implementation of the relational operators may require exhaustive scanning of one or more relations for each retrieval operation, the whole process must be clumsy and expensive with present-day computer architecture and technology.

At Strathclyde we are investigating a general scheme in which a special-purpose processor is used in conjunction with a high-speed random access buffer store and a high-transfer-rate backing store. We believe that this general design has considerable advantages for database work.

## 2. A SPECIAL PURPOSE PROCESSOR

### 2.1 BACKGROUND

Primitive database operations fall into two categories:

(a) Intra record: which can be carried out by referring only to the contents of this record itself (for example simple selection).

(b) Inter record: which require the comparison of the contents of this record with the contents of other records (for example, sorting, merging, joining, projection, division, subtraction, intersection).

In conventional systems the execution speed of both types of operation can be severely limited by the power of the CPU. It is possible to perform some of the above operations by means of a specially extended head-per-track (HPT) associative disk system (Coulouris (1972), Lin (1976), Su). These already offer far higher speeds of operation than systems based on conventional technology. However they lack the generality to perform inter-record operations in a flexible and satisfactory manner.

### 2.2 DESIGN PHILOSOPHY

We have designed and are now constructing a novel form of digital processor (LEECH).

The LEECH processor is a very fast processor capable of carrying out database manipulations. It is attached to the conventional processor which schedules its activities and manipulates the backing stores for it (Figure 2). In some ways therefore, the relationship is analogous to that of an autonomous floating-point processor and a CPU.

The LEECH design takes advantage of the inherently repetitive nature of database operations, in which the same actions must be carried out on each record in a file. It is thus a "natural" vector processor (Figure 3).

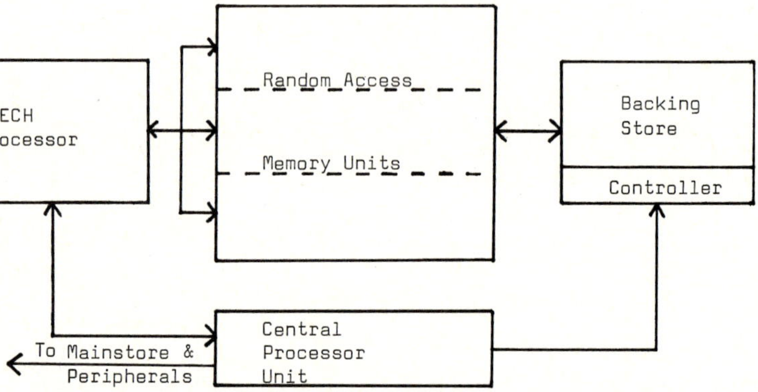


Fig. 2 Architecture of a LEECH based system

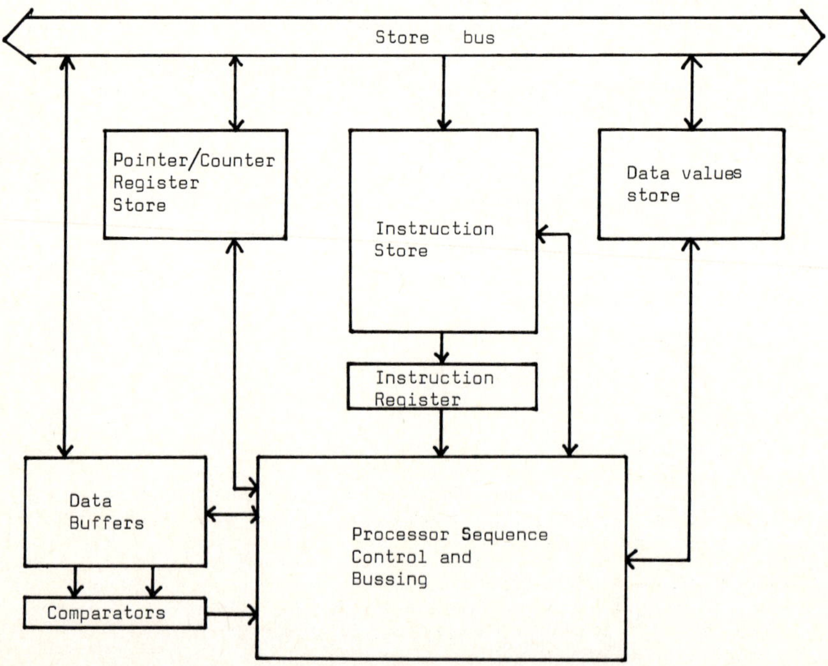


Fig. 3 Internal organisation of LEECH processor

The Random Access Buffer memory may be simply part of the conventional mainstore, or may be high speed memory local to the LEECH itself. Different systems of varying cost/performance ratios may thus be configured to meet the needs of particular applications. The LEECH processor is started by the CPU, and processing of the data in the Buffer Memory then proceeds without further intervention from the CPU. When the operation is complete the LEECH interrupts the CPU. We believe that this organisation possesses several advantages over both conventional and HPT systems.

In particular, LEECH is more efficient than a conventional processor for the following reasons:

1. The LEECH instruction set is specifically tailored for record-oriented operations.

2. The LEECH processor contains a small amount of fast storage space suitable for the storage of instructions. (See Figure 3). Thus, once initialised, LEECH has no need to repeatedly access the host machine's mainstore for instructions. Since, in record-oriented applications, most CPU's require to access at least 10 bytes of instructions for each data byte processed, this technique substantially reduces the load on the mainstore and greatly increases the throughput of the system.

3. LEECH contains a small area of fast storage space suitable for the storage of literal strings, data values and partial results. Thus the mainstore accesses associated with local constants and partial results are eliminated, again reducing the load on the mainstore.

4. A block of registers is provided which may be used as pointers to blocks of data, or as record counters. These would correspond to the accumulators or general registers of a conventional machine, but are more numerous in LEECH, and are dedicated to these functions.

The LEECH will thus process records several orders of magnitude faster than a conventional processor.

The LEECH has the following advantages over HPT systems:

1. Since HPT systems are attached to, and are integral with, some form of rotating mass storage device, the processing operations are normally confined to those which may be performed by serially scanning one information stream. This precludes operations such as merging and similar operations where multiple asynchronous data streams are required. By virtue of its random-access addressing capability, LEECH may perform these operations easily and efficiently.

2. HPT systems are limited in the complexity of the processing algorithms which may be applied to each record as it passes beneath the reading heads. This is due to the fact that the HPT device usually spins continuously at a fixed speed, so that one record's processing must be completed before the next record has been read, in order that the device remain in synchronism with the storage device. This may severely restrict the type of operation which is possible, and/or the performance of the system. If processing is not completed in time the system must wait for one revolution of the HPT device (the latency period) for the record to re-appear in order that processing may continue. In the worst case, the HPT system can incur the latency penalty once per record.

   Our approach removes the need for the record processor to maintain precise synchronism with the storage device by utilising the random-access properties of the Buffer Memory Units. This permits any critical timing effects to be "averaged out" over an entire buffer. Thus if

$n$ = number of records in one buffer

$P_i$ = time taken to process record i

$R_i$ = time taken to read record i from backing store

The HPT systems must satisfy

$$\forall i, P_i < R_i$$

whereas the LEECH need only satisfy the much weaker condition

$$\sum_{i=1}^{i=n} P_i < \sum_{i=1}^{i=n} R_i$$

to prevent latency penalties. In addition, if latency penalties do occur, they only occur once per buffer and not once per record as in HPT systems. Thus system flexibility and performance are improved.

3. Most HPT systems require that the organisation of data on the HPT device be such that reading by multiple heads is facilitated, which usually makes the format of the stored data incompatible with other storage transports. Thus, even though the storage medium may be demountable, it may not be useable on any other transport. The LEECH design contains no such restrictions on data formats.

4. Since HPT systems are integrated with one particular storage device, they may not directly process records residing on another type of device. Our design removes this restriction as the CPU may arrange for any storage device in the system to provide records for processing by LEECH, via the Buffer Memory Units. This produces a more flexible system.

### 2.3 FACILITIES

These are extensible but it is envisaged that the following basic operations will be permanently loaded in the microcode store. The notation used is reasonably straightforward, e.g.

+ denotes logical 'or'

. denotes logical 'and'

EQ denotes the equality relation

literal strings are enclosed in quotes etc.

#### 2.3.1 RECORD SELECTION

(i) Boolean expressions, e.g.

```
NAME EQ 'THOMSON';
NAME EQ 'DAWSON' + NAME EQ 'THOMSON';
AGE GE '19' .AGE LE'25' + NAME EQ 'MACGREGOR';
```

(ii) Inter-field Comparisons, e.g.

NAME1 EQ NAME2 + AGE1 GE AGE2;

(iii) Threshold Function, or "M out of N" expressions, e.g.

(A GE '7', B LT '48', C EQ '1976', D GT '99*'):3;

i.e. if $\geq$ 3 conditions satisfied, we have a hit.

Note that '99*' denotes "any string beginning with '99'" and '*99' would be "any string ending with '99'".

(iv) Weighted Threshold Function, e.g.

(A GE '7'=3, B LT '40'=1, C EQ '1976'=5, D GT '99*'=2):6;

i.e. each condition has a weight associated with it, denoting that term's contribution to the threshold count. If the count equals or exceeds the threshold, we have a hit.

(v) Max/Min Function, e.g.

(a) MAX QTY;

or (b) MAX <FIELD> IN <SELECTION EXPRESSION>;

In case (b) only the records which are hits as defined by the selection expression are eligible for inclusion in the MAX/MIN result.

2.3.2 SORTING

Various sorting algorithms are currently under review and we hope to implement a selection of them in LEECH microcode. Conventional methods of comparing sort algorithms, by evaluating "average number of comparisons" would appear to be largely inapplicable to LEECH, since comparisons may be performed with great speed relative to other operations.

2.3.3 MERGING

Order two, and higher order merges are to be implemented. Although they are faster, high order merges incur larger organisational overheads.

2.3.4 JOIN-MERGE

This instruction performs the equijoin operation, and produces a buffer which contains the join of the contents of two sorted input buffers, over some supplied join field. Note however the alternative algorithms detailed in section 3.

2.3.5 VERTICAL-COMPRESS

This operation eliminates duplicate records from a sorted buffer. Various algorithms are being tested with regard to their speed and ease of implementation within LEECH.

Other operations are being studied, with a view to applications outside of relational databases; these include searching free text, distribution sorts, best fit and pattern matching.

## 2.4 PERFORMANCE ESTIMATES

A small compiler has been written which accepts commands as detailed above. These instructions can then be obeyed by a "LEECH Simulator Program" which simulates LEECH at the register transfer level, and has enabled us to obtain basic timings of various LEECH operations.

Several external factors affect LEECH performance, of which the most important is the speed of the mainstore or buffer store in the host machine. If we opt to attach LEECH to the mainstore (to configure a low cost, but slow system) the simulator shows that a fairly simple selection on one 3330-type disk track of 12½K bytes would take around 500 microseconds. This assumes 800 nS., 16 bit wide store with 80 byte records and a low hit ratio. Under the same conditions, a full sort of a track would take around 40 mS. The use of wider store tends to give an almost linear increase in speed.

For a higher performance system LEECH would be attached to a bipolar Buffer Memory Unit which need not form part of the host machine's address space. The configuration of the store is critical, but by means of long wordlengths, banking and low access times its performance may be increased. When this store is connected to a very high transfer rate backing store, such as a head-per-track disk, drum, CCD or laser store, a very high performance system is created. Our preliminary estimates put the peak searching rate at over 100 Megabytes per second, with performance on the other operations correspondingly improved.

## 2.5 COST

The size of the LEECH machine may be gauged from the fact that it consists of 3 boards, containing the host machine interface, LEECH microprogram store and sequencing kernel, and the LEECH processor, respectively. The high-performance version will require more boards to hold the Buffer Memory Units.

The total component cost of the LEECH prototype has been less than £2,500.

# 3. IMPROVING THE EFFICIENCY OF DATABASE PRIMITIVE OPERATIONS

## 3.1 GENERAL APPROACH

A well-known principle in chemical engineering when refining a mineral ore or similar substance is to use a 2-stage process. The job of the first stage is to extract a "concentrate" from the initial bulk of the crude material, and this "concentrate" is then refined much more precisely to give the final product. Some months ago we discovered new algorithms for relational operations, which use this idea directly.

The principle of the method is to use a fast approximate technique to "filter" the data. This discards a large number of tuples which are not then required to take part in the subsequent stages. The volume of data is also reduced by extracting required fields from tuples, discarding the remainder.

The time taken by the methods is proportional to N the number of tuples handled. No special organisation or prior preparation of the database is required.

In most cases the approximate method must be followed by a further processing stage which ensures that the operation is carried out "strictly". However the second "strict" stage has the advantage of working with a much reduced volume of data.

### 3.2 EQUI-JOIN

The operation of the method is illustrated in Figure 4. The new method requires two fairly large bit-lists. Here we have two relations A (with M tuples) and B (with N tuples). Initially both bit-lists are set to zero. We read in tuples from relation A, say, and hash each join field value to obtain a not-necessarily-unique number, which is used as a bit-list address. We then set the corresponding bit to a '1', irrespective of the value currently in the bit position, and we repeat the operations until we have read all of A and have set a bit to '1' for each tuple. Tuples from A with equal values in their join fields will hash to the same bit-list location. Some non-equal values will hash to the same locations accidentally although a good hashing function will minimise such "accidents".

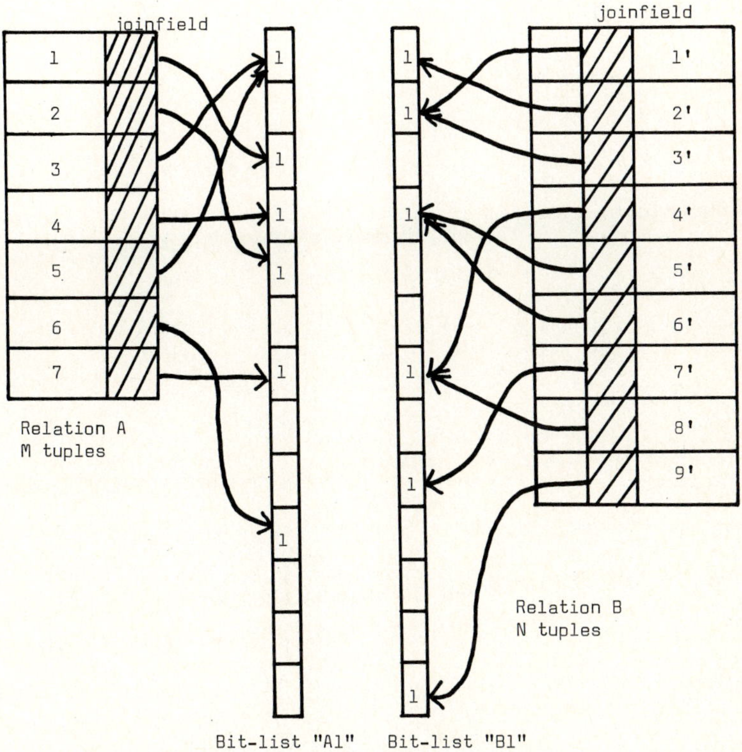


Figure 4 Equi-join, rough selection

Whatever hashing function is used, however, if a bit has not been set to '1' there is no tuple in A with any of the corresponding values.

We read in tuples from relation B, apply the same hashing function to B's join field values, and check the new value against the bit-list constructed for A. Any tuple in B whose join field value hashes to a 'zero' bit on A's bit list will not be needed in the JOIN.

During this pass through B a bit-list can be constructed by hashing the join field values of B tuples which have been shown to be necessary for the join with A. In a similar way, by running through the relation A again, and comparing hash values against B's bit-list we can discard A tuples which are definitely not required in the join. Thus we can obtain two relations A' and B' which generally have fewer tuples than A and B. (In the "worst case" they have the same number of tuples).

It is advantageous to begin by constructing the bit-list of the relation with the smaller number of tuples, then to filter the larger relation against this bit-list. The re-reading of the first relation in order to "filter" it against the second bit-list will take less time when it is the smaller one.

It should be noted that the method is first order with respect to M and N. A' and B' may well contain tuples which do not take part in the join (included because of the non-unique nature of the hashing method). These may well be rejected by subsequent approximate join, projection or intersection operations, or finally when a "strict" method is applied.

The size of bit-list required is limited because -

(i) only one entry per unique value of the join field is required

(ii) even if "overloading" of the bit-list occurs, this merely reduces the efficiency of the filter, but does not invalidate the procedure.

### 3.3 INTERSECTION

The method of carrying out this function is, in its first phase, identical to that described for equi-join.

### 3.4 DIFFERENCE

The difference operation A - B gives a result containing tuples, drawn from A, which do not match any of the tuples in B. The "difference" does not apply to the whole tuple, it only refers to a specified "difference field" in A and B.

We can again use bit-lists to implement the following highly-efficient method.

To subtract relation B (N tuples) from relation A (M tuples) in some specific "difference field" we carry out the following operations:

(i) Form the bit list "B1" for B by hashing the "difference field" values in B.

(ii) Check tuples of A against the bit-list "B1" by "hashing" the A tuple's difference field value.

If the bit is still set to zero, there can be no tuple in B which corresponds to the current A tuple. This tuple is therefore part of the result of A - B and it can be passed out as a result ($C_1$) without further processing. We are then left with a number of A tuples which require more accurate treatment. These form the relation A' with M' tuples, to which we are going to apply a "strict" difference procedure.

(iii) While checking through the A tuples in (b) we construct a new bit-list "A1" corresponding to tuples in A'. The bit-list "A1" can now be used to select members of B which are required for our "strict" difference procedure.

We read through relation B for a second time selecting those tuples whose join-field values match a bit set to '1' in bit-list "A1". These form the smaller relation B' (with N' tuples).

(iv) We must now carry out a "strict" difference operation:

$$C_2 = A'-B'$$

as A' and B' generally have considerably fewer tuples than A and B this can be accomplished rapidly. The overall result C (C=A-B) is

$$C=C_1+C_2$$

(the union of the two partial results).

## 3.5 PROJECTION

The projection operation has two distinct facets -

(i) Extracting the required fields from the tuples of the given relation.

(ii) Ensuring that all tuples of the result are unique i.e. eliminating duplicates from the result.

In suitable cases, a worthwhile acceleration of the second stage can be achieved by using non-unique hashing, in conjunction with bit-lists. A new relation C is to be the result of projecting relation A over the domains y and z. At the first pass through the records representing A, we can extract the appropriate fields to produce a set of records A'. During this pass we hash the entire A' record and obtain a hash-value corresponding to a bit position in bit-lists "A1" and "A2". At the start both bit-lists are initialised to zeros.

We test the bit in "A1" corresponding to the hash value we have obtained for the current record. If this bit is still zero we set it to '1' and take no further action. If, however, it is already set to '1', we have a "collision" and we now must set the corresponding bit in bit-list "A2". On the next pass we "filter" the set of records A' against the bit-list "A2". If a record, when hashed produces a bit-list value for which the bit in bit-list "A2" is zero, then we have a unique record, which requires no further examination. If the bit is set to '1' however the record becomes a member of the set A", which will be subjected to "strict" compression. The result is the union of the two partial results C1 and C2.

## 3.6 RELATIONAL DIVISION

In the following example relation A deals with suppliers and part numbers, while relation B is a set of part numbers. Division of A by B (on part number) gives the set of suppliers who supply all the set of part numbers in B.

| Relation A | | B | A/B |
|---|---|---|---|
| S | P# | P # | S #(=S#P #/P#) |
| A | 1 | 1 | A |
| A | 2 | 2 | C |
| A | 3 | 3 | |
| B | 2 | | |
| B | 3 | | |
| B | 4 | | |
| C | 1 | | |
| C | 2 | | |
| C | 3 | | |
| C | 4 | | |
| D | 5 | | |

Figure 5

The result can be obtained from the sub-set of A which intersects with B on P# . Thus intersection (or an approximate intersection) can be used as an initial pass.

### 3.6.1 APPROXIMATE DIVISION

This would be used as a first pass in order to eliminate most of the data which do not take part in the result of the division. This method follows the same philosophy as the methods already described for join, intersection, difference and projection.

(i) Run through B,hash P#, set corresponding bit in bit-list "B1". Count number of tuples in B (N). Now set up a table "T1" with elements large enough to contain N plus any "accidental" overflow caused by the hashing method. Typically the table would have 8 or 16 bits per entry, depending on N.

(ii) Run through A, hash on P#, if bit in bit-list "B1" is set, hash on S# and increment corresponding count in table "T1". (There is no need to increment this count if it is already greater or equal to N).

(iii) Run through A again, hash on P#, if the bit-list "B1" is set hash on S#, then select the tuple if the table entry in "T1" has a count greater or equal to N. (The "greater than" case is caused by non-unique hashing). The result of this selection is a smaller relation A' which can be checked by a "strict" division method.

### 3.7 OPTIMISATION BY COMBINING APPROXIMATE METHODS

We have indicated earlier that in order to achieve a "strict" result (e.g. projection), a fast approximate stage must be followed by a slower, accurate process. Often, however, a series of approximate operations can be applied one after another without requiring intermediate reprocessing by the slower "strict" methods. This allows scope for considerable optimisation.

Final results must be checked by a "strict" method, of course, and certain operations, such as division, difference and count, must be carried out strictly when they are encountered.

## 3.8 PERFORMANCE OF THE METHODS

Performance is highly data dependent and therefore the effectiveness of the new methods can only be determined in practice. In the "worst case" they amount to an additional overhead, while in a favourable case they can speed up an operation by orders of magnitude. There are, however, general reasons for believing they will prove useful. For instance, as the size of a database increases, a relatively smaller proportion of it is selected to answer an average query. We have tried out some of the methods in actual practice, and results are very encouraging. For example equi-join over all the queries we have given it so far averages x5-x10 better than the unaccelerated method, in terms of tuple I/O transfers. The chief advantages of the new methods are that

(i) they are general, requiring no prior preparation of the data

(ii) they are fast (first order). "Strict" methods are of higher order (N log N) or else require more space than the bit-list methods (e.g. hash-table methods)

(iii) we believe that in suitable systems they will deal with around 90% of the bulk of data handling. We intend to implement the algorithms in the microcode of our special purpose database processor.

## 4. CONCLUSIONS

A minimal prototype of the LEECH processor is now in an advanced state of construction, and is expected to be operational by October 1976. The prototype is attached directly to our department's PDP-11 system, which has conventional disks. Test-bed results from this somewhat limited configuration will then be available to corroborate our simulator predictions. Our initial test system makes use of a database of mass-spectra. In this case we know that the pattern matching required can be done much more rapidly by the LEECH (using the weighted threshold function) than by a conventional processor.

Our investigation of the approximate algorithms is continuing. They will be implemented directly by the LEECH processor.

We believe that our present work shows that not only is a relational database machine a feasible economic proposition, but also that high performance hardware is the key to cost/effective large-scale data-handling.

## 5. ACKNOWLEDGMENTS

We should like to thank the British Science Research Council for support. We should also like to acknowledge the assistance of the staff of ICL's Advanced Research and Development Centre at Stevenage, and in particular E. Babb who first suggested to us bit maps for relational joining operations using a prepared set of values which gave unique bit-list addresses. We have recently become aware that he too had independently discovered the use of bit maps in conjunction with non-unique hashing (Patent Application No. 27093/74) to develop similar methods, which in fact predates some of our work. This work is to be described in a forthcoming paper by Babb. We are grateful to all our colleagues in the Department of Computer Science at the University of Strathclyde for many stimulating discussions.

## 6. REFERENCES

Codd, E.F. (1970) A Relational Model of Data for large shared Databanks (p. 377) CACM Vol. 13, No. 6

Codd, E.F. (1972) Further Normalisation of the Database Relational Model, Database Systems, Courant Computer Science Symposia Series, Vol. 6, Prentice Hall

Coulouris, G.F., Evans, J.M. and Mitchell, R.W. (1972) Towards Content Addressing In Databases (p. 65) Computer Journal, Vol. 15, No. 2 1972

Lin, C.S., Smith, D.C.P. and Smith, J.M. (1976) The Design of a Rotating Associative Memory for Relational Database Applications, TODS, Vol. 1, No. 1

Todd, S. (1975) PRTV A Technical Overview, IBM Report UKSC 0075

Su, S.Y.W., Copland, G.P. and Lipovski, G.P. Retrieval Operations and Data Representations in a Context Addressed Disc System, Department of Electrical Engineering, College of Engineering, University of Florida.

*Systems for Large Data Bases, P.C. Lockemann and E.J. Neuhold, (eds.)*
*North-Holland Publishing Company, 1976*

# AN APPROACH TO DATA COMMUNICATION BETWEEN DIFFERENT GENERALIZED DATA BASE MANAGEMENT SYSTEMS

E. Nahouraii, L. O. Brooks*, and A. F. Cardenas*
International Business Machines Corporation
General Products Division
Palo Alto, California

A number of data base management systems (DBMS) are now in operation in industry, government and the academic world. However, since most of these DBMSs have different conceptual and internal models, they cannot interact and exchange information in a network environment.

This report discusses some of the problems and provides a methodology for communicating and exchanging information between hetrogeneous models of data or DBMSs that are commercially available.

## I. INTRODUCTION

The amount of information stored in machine readable form increases daily. Many firms, realizing the value of their data, have switched from a collection of redundant (and possibly inconsistent) files to a non-redundant, integrated data base or a data base management system (DBMS). Within a firm, the step has meant that previously isolated data, such as marketing file and inventory file data, can now be related. Unfortunately, the individual DBMSs are like their file-oriented predecessors. They are unable to communicate effectively with each other.

As long as different application needs exist and different DBMSs are commercially available, different DBMSs will be used. These systems differ in the logical data base structures that may be defined, what constitutes a data independent query language, access paths provided, how to encode the information, and how to store it physically. For some systems, such as System 2000, a query that is valid at one implementation may not be acceptable at another System 2000 installation which stores the same information with a different logical structure. Furthermore, DBMS-DBMS communication should not significantly degrade the current DBMS operations.

Figure 1 illustrates the essence of the primary problem that we address in this paper: communication between heterogeneous DBMSs, perhaps interconnected in a network environment. Note that two queries are being referred to different systems. Whether the query analyzer directories should be centralized or dispersed will

--------------

*Computer Science Department
University of California, Los Angeles
Los Angeles, California 90024

be discussed later.

Much work has been done on the problem of data conversion by Shoshani, Housel, Lum and Shu (1, 2, 3, 4). These researchers have concentrated on moving the entire data base from one DBMS to another, or from a file management system to a DBMS by defining the data structures of the source and target data. Although concerned with converting data from one system to another, this paper does not address such mass migration of data but rather the communications among different systems to provide an effective information interchange.

Other research activity by Marcus (5) has delt with a translating computer interface for a network of heterogeneous interactive information retrieval systems. However this focuses on the special case of document data bases in which the logical data base structure or user view of the data base is the same; namely, a document. In information retrieval the atomic unit of data access is the "document", whereas in data base management systems the segment or record type, or perhaps each individual field, could be the atomic unit of access. The main differences in the various information retrieval systems is primarly with respect to what access keys or key words are available in the catalog of each document data base.

This paper will interest those considering converting from one DBMS to another. The approach described here makes it possible to use both systems during conversion without having to submit two different (although equivalent) queries, one for each system. Also, if the user has been using a data independent query language, he does not have to change when he upgrades his DBMS.

The next section discusses the various levels at which communication is possible. Section III provides some background on the Data Independent Accessing Model (DIAM) we are using, with particular emphasis on the relevant parts of the model. Section IV explains how we use the model for communication between DBMSs. In Section V, examples of querying different logical structures are walked through. Section VI discusses different logical structures on different DBMSs.

## II. LEVELS OF COMMUNICATION BETWEEN DBMSs

Communication between DBMSs is possible at a variety of levels: a) interactive query level, b) host language level, c) access method level, or d) microscopic level (reading the entire file directly from the storage medium). This last choice burdens a user with the need to know in detail how the system stores data, bypasses most of the system's security controls (e.g., cannot enforce value restricted authorizations), and ignores any access paths (e.g., indexing) that may be available for efficient data retrieval. For these reasons the last choice will not be considered any further.

Communication at one level does not exclude communication at the other levels. Because each query is compiled into access requests, communication at the access request level can provide indirect communication at the query language level. That is, a query is compiled into access requests which, in turn, are translated to other DBMSs. Similarly, a set of access request can be represented by one or more queries; thus, query level communication can be used to translate access requests from one DBMS to another. For linking different DBMSs then, it is desirable to use the level that is most cost effective (in terms of both system resources and user time).

Which level is best? Figure 1 illustrates the various levels. More and more, users know their own system only at the highest level (as a terminal and some high level query language). This implies that communicating at any lower level is impossible due to the limits of the users knowledge, but communicating at this level requires translating a query into other query languages. Even when communicating between two identical DBMS, such as System 2000, a translation may be necessary if the data structures are different, that is, it may be necessary to translate a query into another query in the same language because of restrictions on qualifiers; for example, differences in what keys are inverted to access the data bases. Communication at the access method level can be efficient, but not all users know their own system at this level much less care about how other systems work. Our solution, developed later in this paper, combines the query level with the access method level to take advantage of the benefits of both: high level for user convenience and access-path level for better efficiency.

It is interesting to note that in a number of systems like IMS and DBTG, the data accessing language (DL/1, DML) is designed for a logical structure (hierarchy, network) which corresponds rather directly to the access path storage structure. Thus, the translation problem from the host language level to the access method level is perhaps not so complex. However, the translation problem from the interactive query level to a lower level is complex. The problem is complex and one needs more general methods when there is not a close correspondence of the structures on different levels. This is the case when communicating across different systems, so one needs to introduce a more complex translation process.

Various ways of characterizing DBMS exist. Most vendors give a two-tier view - an upper "logical" level for the user and a proprietary level. Many researchers in data base system structure have used three levels of data description: external model (user or application program logical view), data base model (schema) and internal model (physical and storage). With these divisions, the logical level usually encompasses the logical structure (e.g., hierarchy), as well as the purely logical aspects of the data. In some systems the data base model level includes file indexing, access paths within files, and inversion capabilities. Because the path from a main segment to its subsegments falls into both the logical and storage levels, the better resolution of the Data Independent Accessing Method (DIAM) (6, 7, 8) is needed to avoid this confusion. (The full generality of DIAM introduces more detail than we need, so we use only those parts that benefit us).

## III. THE DIAM FRAMEWORK

DIAM provides four successive levels of abstraction: 1) entity set model, 2) string model, 3) encoding model, and 4) physical device level model. Each level may be combined with the higher levels to characterize a DBMS at any level of machine dependency. The entity set model represents the information stored about an object with no regard to how this information is stored or presented to the user; it is purely a logical view of the data base. See for example the Employee and Department entities in Figure 2. The string model describes access paths in terms of connected, ordered subsets of the information contained in the entities. A string is

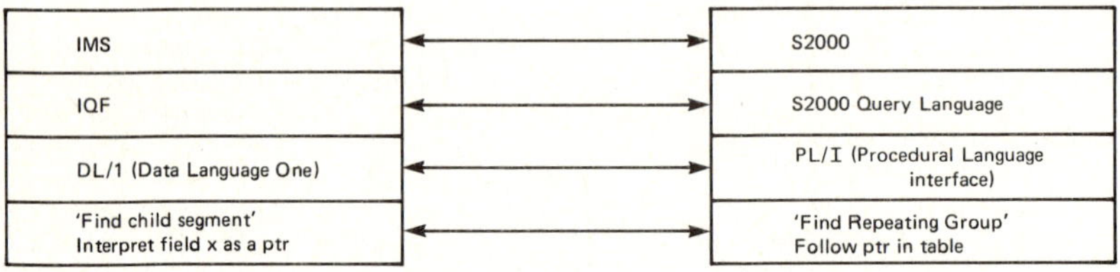


Figure 1. Communication levels between two systems.

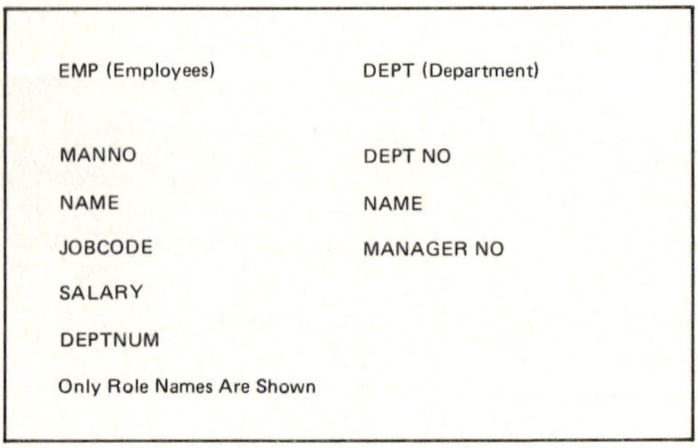


Figure 2. Entity sets for language example.

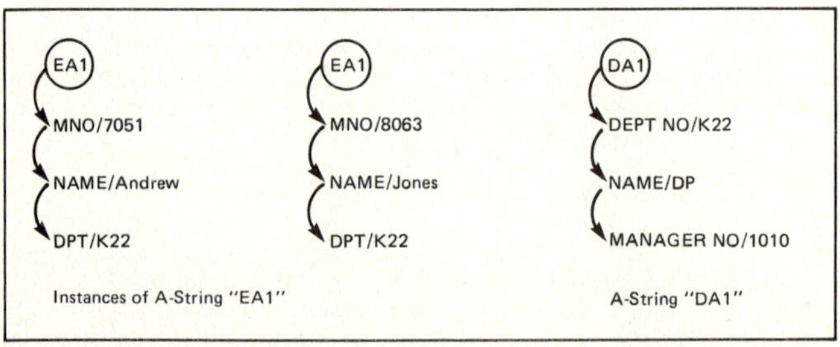


Figure 3. A-string instances.

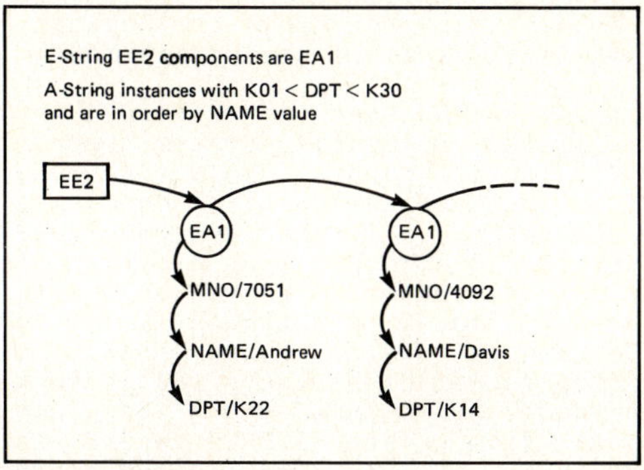


Figure 4. E-string.

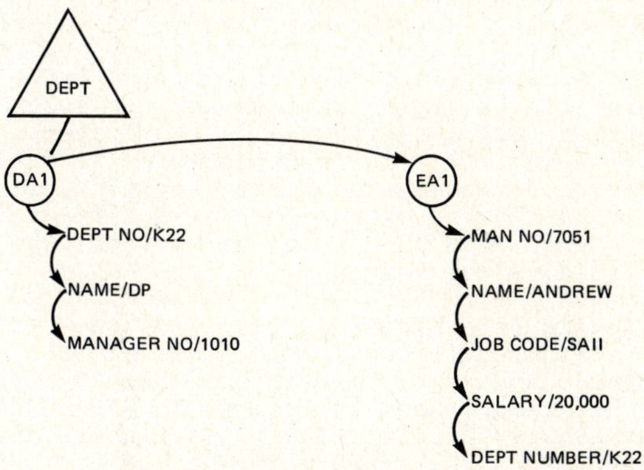


Figure 5. A DIAM L-string connecting one DEPT entity with an employee entity based on a match in DEPT NO.

specified by the elements on the string, their order, and the strings to which the given string connects. The encoding model describes the bit level encoding of the strings in a general way. The physical device level deals with the subdivision of physical devices into blocks and/or tracks, etc., as well as the mapping of the linear address spaces into the physical device. In particular, the related concepts of logical data structure and data accessing paths have been brought together from the logical and storage levels into their own level, that of the string model.

The string model can be used to provide a system independent characterization of the necessarily system-dependent access paths into the data. More to the point, the string model presents a favorable tradeoff of standardization (for communication) and system dependence (for efficiency). The string model describes a file in terms of three types of strings. An A-string (ASG) connects a specified subset of attributes of a single entity in a specified order. See Figure 3. Thus a conventional file record, DBTG record type, and an IMS segment may be represented. An E-string (ESG) connects a specified subset of elements that have the same A-string structure or type description in a specified order. See Figure 4. Thus a conventional file, a set of DBTG record occurrences, and a set of IMS segment occurrences may be represented. An L-string (LSG) connects elements (which may be an A-string, E-string, or another L-string) based on the value of one attribute which occurs in each element. See Figure 5. Thus an L-string may represent a DBTG set and an IMS segment hierarchy.

The strings are described in a string catalog which contains the string name, its type, and its parameters. The parameters are comprised of an element list (EXL), the elements (in order) on the string, how the string is composed, and on which strings the given string is an element. A section of string is defined by selecting two elements on a string; the first (in string order) is considered as the beginning of the string section and the second is called the end of the section (e.g., in figure 4, EE2 connecting only the two EA1 instances shown). It is then possible to define a (string) path as a connected sequence of string sections, i.e., the end of one section is the beginning of the next. Generally, a user is interested in a path from one set of attributes (the qualifiers) to another (the field values sought).

String skipping is defined as following one string to an element on that string, but then leaving that element by following a different string. An example of string skipping, in terms of Figure 4, is the procedure used to locate the DEPARTMENT (DPT) of an employee named Davis; the EE2 string is traversed to the correct EA1 string (NAME = DAVIS) then "skipping" to the EA1 string which is followed to attribute DEPARTMENT. In conventional terms, the above operation is described as consulting the name index to locate the correct record, and then the department field is examined. Note that, in the DIAM formulation, the specific access mechanisms of the system (necessary to identify Davis' department) have been identified without making any assumptions about their implementation, that is, EA1 may be physical contiguity, pointers, or some other method of relating those fields into the record (entity).

String switching is defined as following an A-string to some attribute on that A-string but them switching to a different entity (and hence different A-string) based on a match of the arrribute value. In terms of Figure 5, it is possible to follow EA1 to DEPT

NUMBER but then switch to DA1 and proceed to MANAGER NO. This procedure is very similar to finding the JOIN of two distinct types of tuples in the relational approach. Note that if the attribute used for switching is not a key field in the second A-string, the switching can be very time consuming. Also, in general, switching in the reverse direction (DA1 to EA1) can result in several EA1 instances since usually a department will contain more than one employee. By application of string switching (and shifting) the string model also serves to identify what information may be obtained from the data base through iterative questioning. When a user asks a sequence of questions and the result of each question is used as a search criterion for the next question, he is said to be iteratively querying the data base. Consider Figure 2. Although there is no direct string path from MAN NUMBER to manager's salary (in fact, there is not even a field defined as manager's salary), an employee can query his own record to obtain DEPARTMENT NUMBER (DEPTNUM), then query the department file to obtain MANAGER NUMBER, and finally query the employee file to obtain his manager's record (including salary). Note that this information is not directly (one query) available but may be obtained by iterative querying.

What has happened is that equivalence classes have been defined; DEPARTMENT NUMBER in EMPLOYEE has been identified with DEPARTMENT NUMBER iN DEPARTMENT. Thus, the string EA1, Figures 3 or 5, is traversed to DEPARTMENT NUMBER; the user then switches to the string DA1, i.e., he reenters the data base to the instance of DA1 where DEPARTMENT NUMBER equals the DEPARTMENT NUMBER returned in the previous query. String DA1 is followed to MANAGER NUMBER. Here, a second equivalence class relating MANAGER NUMBER and MAN NUMBER is created and the user switches to another instance of E1 (his manager's) and follows that to SALARY. In designing data base security, this model serves to highlight where extra protection is needed to limit the information that can be collected by iterative queries.

## IV. APPROACH TO COMMUNICATION BETWEEN HETEROGENEOUS DBMSs

The string model of a DBMS represents the paths into and through the data stored by that DBMS. The strings are defined by the Data Base Administrator (DBA) when he selects a data structure and index values. Note that the strings already exist for a given data base in the DBMS and are, in fact, used by the DBMS to answer queries. The technique for connecting heterogeneous DBMSs is that each DBMS be required to maintain a DIAM string catalog (augmented by a table defining how to traverse each type of string). See figure 6. Each DBMS continues to operate exactly as before; that is, no internal changes are required.

To query another DBMS, a user submits his query as usual on his own DBMS; but this time as the query is analyzed for which attributes must be examined, a string path in the second DBMS is constructed to connect these attributes. Where is this path constructed? If a centralized approach (i.e., a central repository for all the string catalogs) is chosen, then that is where the path would probably be constructed. If a decentralized network structure is chosen, then each node maintains its own string catalog and the path may be constructed at either the questioning or answering node depending on which is the less expensive node. A more detailed analysis is carried out by W. Chu and E. Nahouraii (9) on the cost function at each, i.e., the query may be analyzed against the available strings at either node but presumably this will be done at the less expensive node.

Since there may be more than one string path, the speed (cost) of traversing each string should be included in the catalog. This allows optimal string path selection and improves network utilization. If all nodes are equally likely to contain the desired information, then searching should begin with the least expensive node since, in general, half the nodes must be searched.

## V. ILLUSTRATIONS OF COMMUNICATION BETWEEN DIFFERENT DATA STRUCTURES

The following examples show communication between different data structures on the same DBMS. Later, we extend the ideas developed here to communication between different types of DBMSs. System 2000 (10) is used due to the straightforwardness of its DDL and data structure. Other hierarchical systems will have similar string catalogs (because the underlying data structures are similar). The main difference will be in the cost associated with each type of string traversal. Some systems will provide more strings and others less, but since the problem illustrated here is communication between different logical structures, three different structures on System 2000 provide enough relevant differences to begin with.

An airline, for example, will want to store information about its planes and its passengers. Three possible ways to structure the information are shown in Figure 7. The first case (SI) structures its data to consist of a record for each plane and associates with each plane record several passenger records. The second (SII) maintains a collection of passenger records, part of which is plane/flight information. Note that there is considerable duplication of plane information -- the plane fields are identical for all passengers on the same plane. The third approach consists of a set of location records and associates with each airport a number of plane records and a number of passenger records. In this case, given a passenger name, two accesses must be made to determine his destination: First, find the PLANE IDEN for the passenger and then use that as PLANE IDEN to find the DEST. This is string switching.

The string models of SI, SII, and SIII are shown in Figures 8, 9, and 10, respectively. The respective string catalogs are in Figures 11, 12, 13, but the following discussion will be easier to follow by using Figures 8, 9, and 10. As Figure 8 is compared with SI in Figure 7, the question arises as to why PLANE ID is included in the passenger entity (Figure 8) but not in the PASSENGERS segment (Figure 7). The reason is that it is implicitly included by virtue of PASSENGERS being a subsegment of the PLANE segment. The PLANE ID is present in the PASSENGER record in some form (perhaps physical placement or pointer). This is an advantage to the string model because <u>all</u> information stored must be explicitly identified.

Figure 8 shows the fields of the PLANE segment connected by an A-string; similarly, the fields of the passenger segment are connected by Y. An E-string, PASS ON PLANE, connects all the passengers on a given plane; it is partitioned by PLANE ID, i.e., for

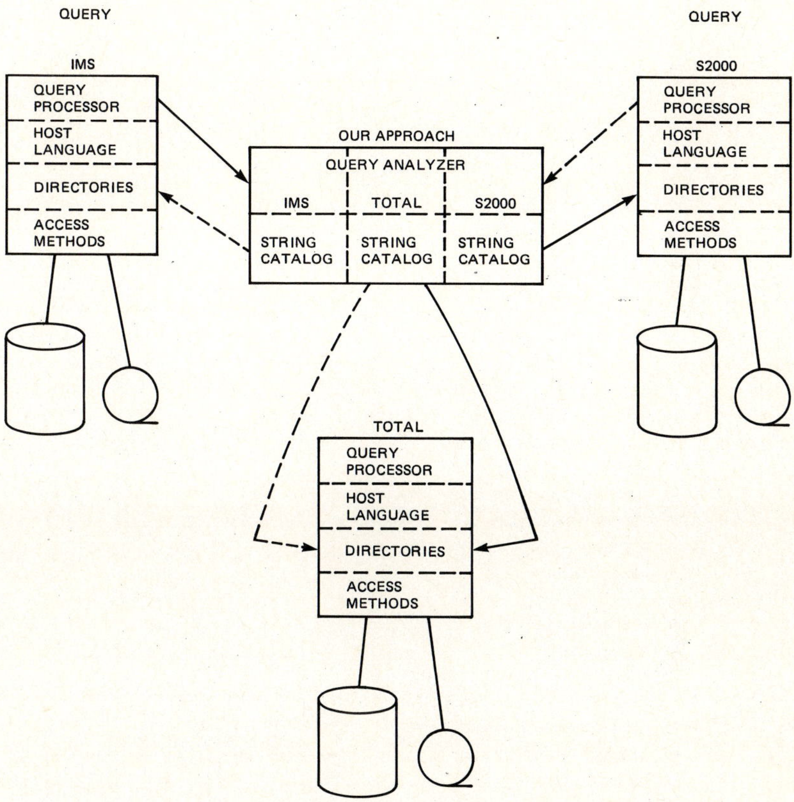


Figure 6. Our approach is the central box composed of query analyzers and string catalogs. The solid arrows show the path of a query entered on an IMS installation (via IQF) to the other systems that need to be queried. The dotted arrows show a query entered on S2000. The path of query entered on TOTAL is not shown to keep the figure simple.

SI

1. PLANE ID (NAME X(10))
2. TYPE (NON-KEY NAME X(5))
3. LOC (KEY NAME X(3))
4. FLT NO (NON-KEY NAME X(5))
5. DEST (KEY NAME X(3))
6. PASSENGERS (RG)
7. SEAT ID (NON-KEY) NAME IN6 X(4))
8. PASS NAME (KEY NAME IN6 X (10))
9. ADDRESS (NON-KEY NAME IN6 X(15))

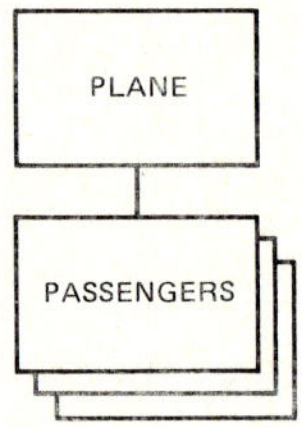


SII

1. PASS NAME (KEY NAME X(10))
2. ADDRESS (NON-KEY NAME X(15))
3. SEAT ID (NON-KEY NAME X(4))
4. PLANE ID (KEY NAME X(10))
5. TYPE (NON-KEY NAME X(5))
6. LOC (KEY NAME X(3))
7. FLT NO (NON-KEY NAME X(5))
8. DEST (KEY NAME X(3))

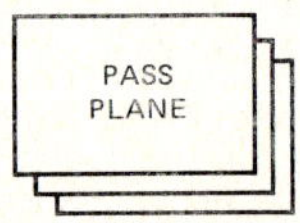


SIII

1. LOC (KEY NAME X(3))
2. PLANES (RG)
3. PLANE ID (KEY NAME INZ X(10))
4. TYPE (NON-KEY NAME INZ X(5))
5. FTL NO (NON-KEY NAME INZ X (5))
6. DEST (KEY NAME IN2 X(3))
7. PASSENGERS (RG)
8. SEAT ID (NON-KEY NAME IN7 X(4))
9. PASS NAME (KEY NAME IN7 X(10))
10. ADDRESS (NON-KEY NAME IN7 X(15))
11. PLANE IDEN (KEY NAME IN7 X(10))

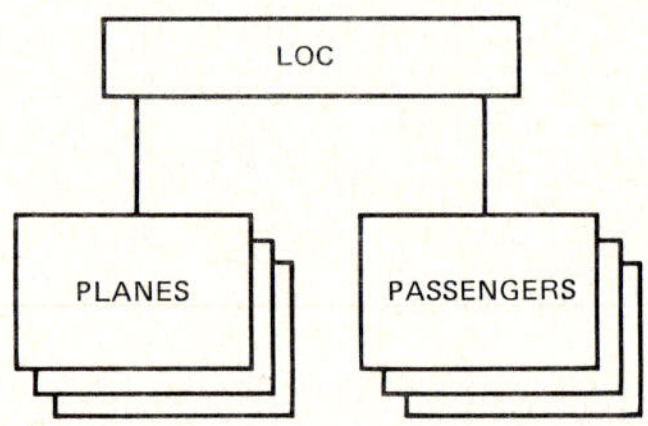


Figure 7. Three possible logical ways to define an airline passengers data base in S2000.

each distinct PLANE ID in the passenger entities, there is an instance of the E- string PASS ON PLANE connecting all passenger entities with (on) the same PLANE ID.

In reality, this E-string would probably be ordered on SEAT, but the example is to show the strings and not a complete data base for an airline. The hierarchy (PLANE is a main segment to PASSENGER) is shown in the L-string flight; it connects a plane with the passengers on the plane. The PASS PLANE L-string is included to show that the user can go from a subsegment to a main segment. The E-strings AIRPLANE ID, LOCATION, DESTINATION, and NAMES denote indexes (keys) into the data base.

The main question in Figure 10 is why two L-strings are used to represent the hierarchy instead of one L-string connecting a PLANES AT LOCATION and PASS AT LOCATION. Both approaches, one or two L-strings, have the same access possibilities. Neither has fewer fields connected; but the storage structure of S2000 is more closely reflected by the two string approach. In any event, the approach used is irrelevant to the following discussion.

Consider the query "LIST ALL PASSENGERS ON PLANE ABC" by tracing it to see how it is answered for each of the three structures in Figure 7. Looking at Figure 8, SI answers this command by consulting the plane index to locate the record plane ABC; then the system examines each child (passenger) segment associated with this plane record. This process, locating all the passenger records of passengers on plane ABC, will now be described in terms of the string model. The E-string AIRPLANE ID is used to locate the record (A-string x) where PLANE ID = ABC, since it is ordered on PLANE ID; the user then follows the FLIGHT L-string to the collection of passengers on plane ABC (i.e., the E-string PASS ON PLANE). This E-string is traversed printing the name in each passenger record on it.

Figures 7 (SI) and 8 show the path that the E-string AIRPLANE ID follows to the instances of the A-string x, where PASS PLANE = ABC and then prints the passenger name. Informally, SII consults the AIRPLANE ID index to locate all records where the PASS PLANE field is ABC.

Note that the right half of Figure 10 is similar to Figure 8. In particular the AIRPLANE NUMBER string (which corresponds to AIRPLANE ID in Figure 8) is followed to the appropriate A-string E, and the passenger names are printed.

What has the string model given us? In the above paragraph, it was used to provide a formalized description of which access paths a particular system needs to use to answer a given query. "Passing from a parent segment to its children segments" may be adequate description for hierarchical systems to communicate but then, if the underlying data structure is a network or a relation, it probably is not sufficiently well defined.

If each DBMS maintains a table of how the strings are implemented, a sequence of string paths can be converted into specific access requests on a given DBMS regardless of the data structure used by that DBMS. The string model gives us an intermediate level between the query language and the access mechanisms which allows us to utilize both in the network. A query is compiled into a string path which is translated into specific access requests; thus

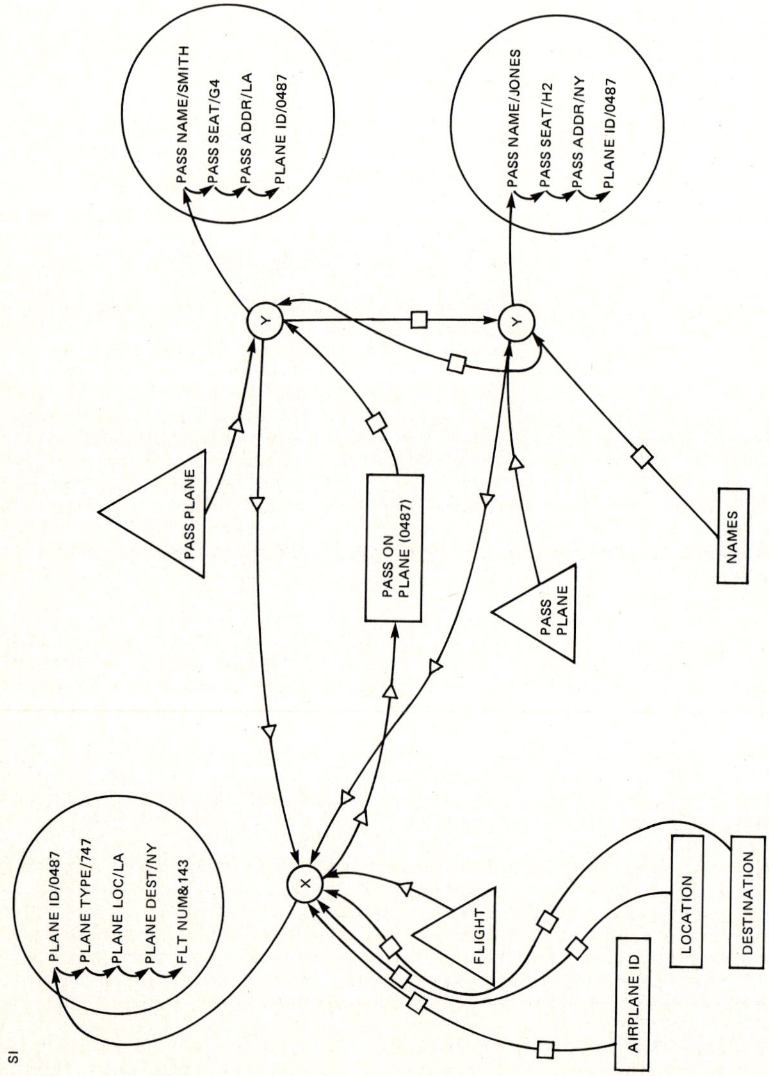


Figure 8. The string model for one plane entity and two associated passengers.

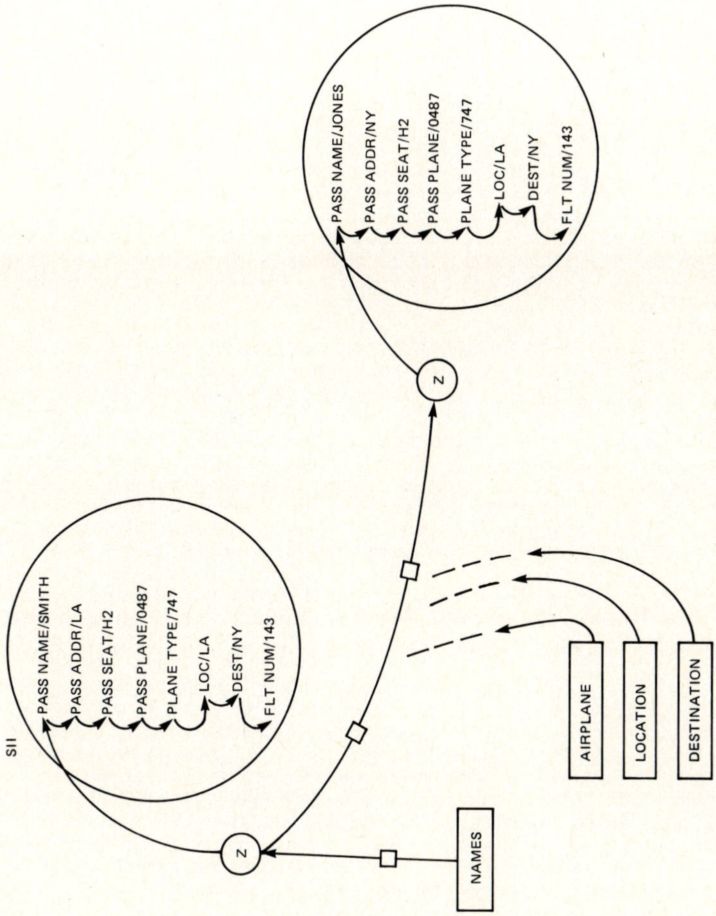


Figure 9. String model for two passenger entities.

both the query language, striving to minimize user time, and the access mechanisms, striving to minimize machine time, are used.

A second query is given to illustrate further. Suppose a user with the data base view SI in Figure 7 types in the query "LIST DESTINATION WHERE PASS NAME = SMITH." On his own system, this query is dealt with as usual by System 2000 but for illustration, the string solution is included. The name index (E-string NAMES) is followed to all instances of passengers name Smith, from each such record, the PASS PLANE L-string is used to locate the plane record associated with the passenger name Smith; then the A-string A is followed to the DESTINATION ATTRIBUTE. This is described in conventional terms as using the name index to locate all records of passengers name Smith and then examining the parent (PLANE) segments for the destinations.

How will our DIAM Catalog accomplish this? There are two parts to the query: 1) how to identify the subset qualified by the query and 2) how to pass from that subset to the desired attribute(s). The first part deals with selecting a subset of the data base; it is here that the indexing (E-strings) are used to determine what portion of the data base we wish to restrict ourselves to or, conversely, how much sequential processing must be done. The second part deals with interpreting the DDL which is possible for heterogeneous types of DBMS only if some standard form for the relationships of attributes is used. In other words, the isolation of the accessing paths and data structure into the String Model provides enough information to answer queries without any extraneous material.

If the query "LIST DESTINATION WHERE PASSNAME = SMITH" failed to return any information in the previous paragraph, the user may want to check the records of the other airlines using the data base structures SII and SIII, Figure 7. The first task for our machinery is to examine the data bases to see how to locate those records of passengers named Smith. The second part of answering the query is the construction of a path from passenger name to his plane's destination. In practice, this will be done in terms of searching the catalog in Figures 12 and 13, but the reader new to DIAM may find it easier to follow the discussion using Figures 9 and 10.

What A-strings are the attributes on? For Figure 8, PASSenger NAME is on Y and PLANE DESTination is on X; so now the problem is reduced to finding a path from Y to X. Such a path may be constructed either from Y to X, by finding a string segment from Y ending "closer" to X, a string segment from there ending even closer to X, until one is found that ends at X or by finding a path which ends at X, a path to where that path begins, ..., even a path from Y to where that path begins, i.e., a path may be constructed in either a forward or backward manner. In this example, we find PASSenger PLANE (an L-string, child segment to parent) from Y to X, though in a more complicated example, it may be necessary to construct a sequence of paths. So, in summary, the final resolution is that we use NAMES to locate each passenger named Smith and then use the strings PASSenger PLANE and X to arrive at the destination.

Before proceeding further, it is necessary to ask if the above paragraphs describe how a real DBMS answers a query. If one considers what is done by the DBMS only at a purely logical level, the answer is yes; but most DBMSs take advantage of storage considera-

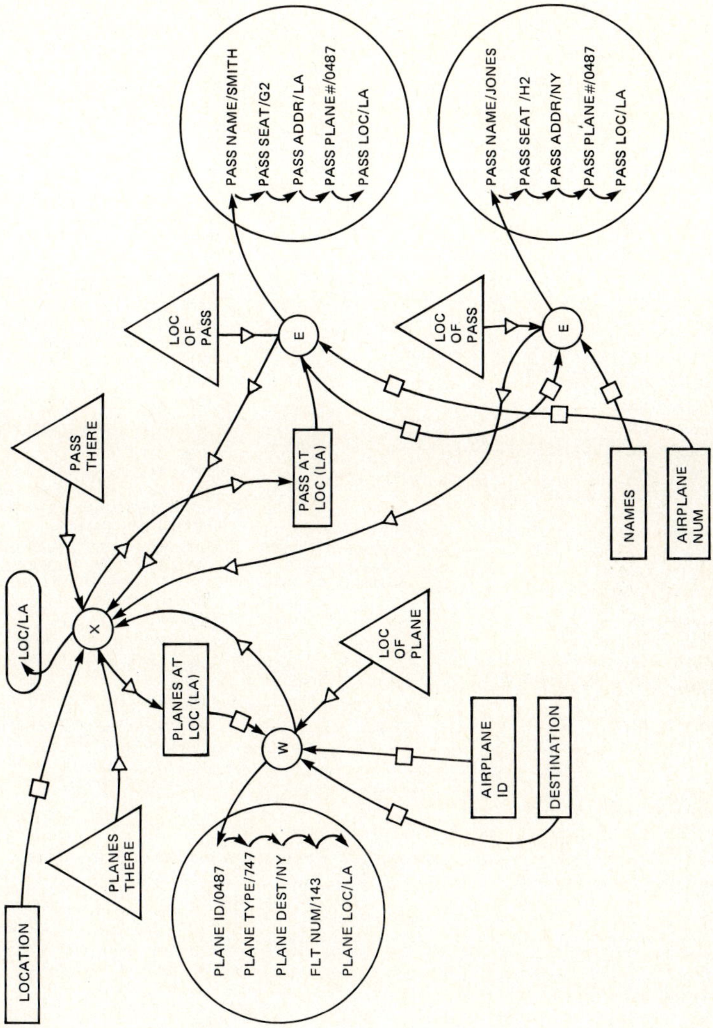


Figure 10. String model for one location entry, one plane entry and two passenger entries.

| NAME | TYPE | IDENTIFIERS | STRING NAME | STRING TYPE | STRING PARAMETERS |
|---|---|---|---|---|---|
| PLANE | DSN | (PLANE ID, LOC, DEST) | X | ASG | [EXL = (PLANE ID, PLANE TYPE, PLANE LOG, PLANE DEST, FLT NUM); ON = FLIGHT; ON = LOCATION; ON = DESTINATION; ON = AIRPLANE ID] |
| | | | LOCATION | ESG | [EXL = 00 = (X LOC); ON = ENTRY] |
| | | | DESTINATION | ESG | [EXL = 00 = (X DEST); ON = ENTRY] |
| | | | AIRPLANE ID | ESG | [EXL = X; 00 = (X ID); ON = ENTRY] |
| | | | FLIGHT | LSG | [EXL = X, PASS ON PLANE); MOC = (X PLANE ID = Y PLANE); ON = AIRPLANE ID] |
| PLANE ID | RN | -- | -- | -- | [ON = X] |
| PLANE TYPE | RN | -- | -- | -- | [ON = X] |
| PLANE LOC | RN | -- | -- | -- | [ON = X] |
| PLANE DEST | RN | -- | -- | -- | [ON = X] |
| FLT NUM | RM | -- | -- | -- | [ON = X] |
| PASS | DSN | (NAME) | -- | ASG | [EXL = (PASS NAME, PASS SEAT, PASS ADDR, PASS PLANE); ON = (PASS ON PLANE); ON = (NAMES)] |
| | | | PASS ON PLANE | ESG | [EXL = Y; PART = (Y PLANE); 00 = (PASS SEAT); ON = (FLIGHT)] |
| | | | NAMES | ESG | [EXL = Y; 00 = (Y PASS NAME); ON = ENTRY] |
| PASS NAME | RN | -- | -- | -- | [ON = Y] |
| PASS SEAT | RN | -- | -- | -- | [ON = Y] |
| PASS ADDR | RN | -- | -- | -- | [ON = Y] |
| PASS PLANE ID | RN | -- | -- | -- | [ON = Y] |
| | | | PASS PLANE | LSG | [EXL (Y, X); MC = (Y PLANE = X PLANE ID); ON = ENTRY] |

Figure 11. String catalog for plane passenger DB with logical structure of SI in Figure 7 and string model in Figure 8.

tions. In the above example, finding the destination of a given passenger, in Figure 7, the system "KNOWS" from the DDL that destination is stored in the main segment to passenger and so does not have to construct explicitly the path from name to destination that it uses to answer the query. Already mentioned is the reduction in storage space by not including PLANE ID in the PASSENGERS segment, Figure 7, SI, by incorporating it into the hierarchy.

Similar assumptions and "tricks" make a DBMS faster than if string paths must be explicitly constructed. But these assumptions and tricks will not work where the underlying structure upon which they are based is not known (as in a network of a heterogeneous DBMS). A DBMS may make assumptions and utilize whatever techniques it chooses in implementing the interpretation of the command to follow a particular string; this is where much efficiency over the full DIAM can be realized.

Back to the command "LIST DESTINATION WHERE PASS NAME = SMITH". As shown in figures 9 and 12, the model already has an A-string Z leading from NAME to DESTination, so that the needed path is already there. What remains to be done is to extract the correct subset. The E-string NAMES, ordered on PASS NAME, facilitates quick selection of the correct subset, i.e., binary search of the inverted name values. In other words, we use the NAMES index to locate passenger records where PASS NAME = SMITH and then examine the DESTINATION field.

Figures 10 and 13 present more difficulty in constructing a path from PASS NAME to the DESTINATION of the plane that the passenger is using. Again, we use the E-string NAMES (the name index) to locate the correct subset. But to traverse from the PASSENGER NAME field to the right DESTINATION field, we must follow the LOCATION OF PASSENGERS (parent) L-string to S and then the PLANES THERE (child) L-string to PLANES AT LOCATION (twins E-string). Then each W on PLANES AT LOCATION must be tested for a match of W. PLANE ID with E. PLANE NUMBER.

Is this the best we can do? No. When selecting the minimal cost path, string switching must also be considered. The string switching solution involves realizing that the fields W PLANE ID with E. PLANE NUMBERS are to be matched (as must be done anyway) so that we can go from PASSENGER NAME (search criterion) to PLANE NUMBER and from PLANE ID to DESTINATION (desired information), and that PLANE ID is indexed by AIRPLANE ID (an E-string). Thus, the string switching solution merely has to locate the passenger for PASS NAME = SMITH and then take PLANE NUMBER as a search criterion in the plane files. When Smith's plane is found, the DESTINATION fields can be examined. What if the plane records were not indexed by AIRPLANE ID? Then the first approach restricts the portion of the plane file that must be examined to those planes at the same airport as Smith, certainly much better than searching the entire set of plane records.

All the previous discussion in this section also apply similarly to other DBMS'. Note that the System 2000 structures in Figure 7 are equivalent to the following normalized relational data base structures:

Structure S1:

AIRPLANES(<u>PLANE ID</u>,TYPE,LOC,FLT NO,DEST)

| NAME | TYPE | IDENTIFIERS | STRING NAME | STRING TYPE | STRING PARAMETERS |
|---|---|---|---|---|---|
| PASSENGER | DSN | (PASS NAME, PASS PLANE, LOC, DEST) | Z | ASG | [EXL = (PASS NAME, PASS ADDR, PASS SEAT, PASS PLANE, TYPE LOC, DEST, FLT NUM); ON = NAMES; ON = AIRPLANE ID; ON = LOCATION, ON = DESTINATION) |
| | | | NAMES | ESG | [EXL = (Z); 00 = (PASS NAME); ON = ENTRY] |
| | | | AIRPLANE IE | ESG | [EXL = (Z); 00 = (Z PASS PLANE); ON = ENTRY] |
| | | | LOCATION | ESG | [EXL = (Z); 00 = (Z LOC); ON = ENTRY] |
| | | | DESTINATION | ESG | [EXL = (Z); 00 = (Z DEST); ON = ENTRY] |
| PASS NAME | RN | -- | -- | -- | [ON = Z] |
| PASS ADDR | RN | -- | -- | -- | [ON = Z] |
| PASS SEAT | RN | -- | -- | -- | [ON = Z] |
| PASS PLANE | RN | -- | -- | -- | [ON = Z] |
| PLANE TYPE | RN | -- | -- | -- | [ON = Z] |
| LOC | RN | -- | -- | -- | [ON = Z] |
| DEST | RN | -- | -- | -- | [ON = Z] |
| FLT NUM | RN | -- | -- | -- | [ON = Z] |

Figure 12. String catalog for plane passenger DB with logical structure of SII in Figure 7 and string model in Figure 9.

| NAME | TYPE | IDENTIFIERS | STRING NAME | STRING TYPE | STRING PARAMETERS |
|---|---|---|---|---|---|
| LOC | DSN | (LOC) | S | ASG | [EXL = (LOC); ON = LOCATION; ON = PLANES THERE; ON = PASS THERE; ON = LOC OF PLANE; ON = LOC OF PASS] |
| | | | LOCATION | ESG | [EXL = (S); 00 = (LOC); ON = ENTRY] |
| | | | PLANES THERE | LSG | [EXL = (S, PLANES AT LOC); MC = (S LOC = W LOC); ON = ENTRY] |
| | | | PASS THERE | LSG | [EXL = (S, PASS AT LOC); MC = (S LOC = E LOC); ON = ENTRY] |
| PLACE/LOC | RN | –– | –– | –– | [ON = S] |
| PLANE | DSN | (PLANE ID, DEST) | W | ASG | [EXL = (PLANE ID, P TYPE, P DEST, FLT NUM, P. LOC); ON = PLANES AT LOC; ON = LOC OF PLANE] |
| | | | PLANES AT LOC | ESG | [EXL = (S); PART = (W LOC) ON = PLANES THERE] |
| | | | LOC OF PLANES | LSG | [EXL = (W, S); MC = (W LOC = S LOC); ON = AIRPLANE ID; ON = ENTRY |
| | | | AIRPLANE ID | ESG | [EXL = W); 00 = (PLANE ID); ON = ENTRY] |
| | | | DESTINATION | ESG | [EXL = W); 00 = (DEST); ON = ENTRY] |
| PLANE ID | RN | –– | –– | –– | [ON = (W)] |
| PLANE TYPE | RN | –– | –– | –– | [ON = (W)] |
| PLANE DEST | RN | –– | –– | –– | [ON = (W)] |
| FLT NUM | RN | –– | –– | –– | [ON = (W)] |
| PLANE LOC | RN | –– | –– | –– | [ON = (W)] |
| PASSENGER | DSN | (PASS NAME, PASS PLANE NUM) | E | ASG | [EXL = (PASS NAME, PASS SEAT, PASS ADDR, PASS PLANE NUM, PASS LOC); ON = PASS AT LOC; ON = LOC OF PASS] |
| | | | PASS AT LOC | ESG | [EXL = (E); PART = (E LOC); ON = PASS THERE] |
| | | | LOC OF PASS | LSG | [EXL = (E, S); MC = (E LOC) = S LOC); ON = ENTRY] |
| | | | NAMES | ESG | [EXL = (E); 00 = (PASS NAME); ON = ENTRY] |
| | | | AIRPLANE NUM | ESG | [EXL = (E); 00 = (PASS LOC); ON = ENTRY] |
| PASS NAME | RN | –– | –– | –– | [ON = E] |
| PASS SEAT | RN | –– | –– | –– | [ON = E] |
| PASS ADDR | RN | –– | –– | –– | [ON = E] |
| PASS PLANE NUM | RN | –– | –– | –– | [ON = E] |
| PASS LOC | RN | –– | –– | –– | [ON = E] |

Figure 13. String catalog for plane passenger DB with logical structure of SIII in Figure 7 and string model in Figure 10.

PASSENGERS (PLANE ID,SEAT ID,PASS NAME,ADDRESS)

Structure S2:

PASS (PASS NAME,ADDRESS,SEAT ID,PLANE ID,TYPE,LOC,
FLT NO,DEST)

Structure S3:

LOCATION(LOC)
LOCPLANES(LOC,PLANES,PLANE ID,TYPE,FLT NO,DEST)
LOCPASSENGERS(LOC,SEAT ID,PASS NAME,ADDRESS,PLANE IDEN)

## VI. COMMUNICATION BETWEEN DIFFERENT DBMSs

The previous section illustrated communication between different logical structures on the same DBMS (System 2000). What happens if the communicating systems are different types of DBMSs? Figure 14a gives a simplified DBD generation or schema description of an IMS (11) data base for the airline information. Figure 14b represents that structure pictorially. Note that the parent information is explicit in the child segment definition, but implicit in System 2000. The string model is essentially the same as Figure 8; the primary difference is the addition of several E-strings which make it possible to traverse several of the E-strings in Figure 8 (e.g., PASS ON PLANE) in reverse order.

Because the string model of the IMS data base generated in Figure 14a contains the string model of System 2000 (Figure 8) as a subset, that discussion on answering the example queries still holds. There may be a better (faster and/or cheaper) path, but at this stage we are showing feasibility. The similarity of the catalogs of IMS and System 2000 is the reason we selected the string model. It provides a convenient standard in which to express access paths whether they are explicitly defined by the DBA or implicitly defined by the logical data structure.

Up to this point, we have only considered hierarchical systems. As an example of a nonhierarchical data base, we will express the airline information in TOTAL (12). Figure 15 gives the declaration of our data base in TOTAL as a plane file and passenger file connected by the APLA file. The data structure is shown in Figure 16. In TOTAL, it is possible to associate several planes with one passenger without duplicating the passenger record as must be done in System 2000.

Figure 17 shows the string model. Note that since airplanes and passengers can now be associated in a many-to-many relationship, the association is an entity in itself. For the first query, listing all passengers on a given plane, the AIRPLANE ID index is used to locate the names. The second query, find destination for a given passenger, requires that the NAME index be used to locate all planes that the passenger is on and then following the LINK TO PLANE RECORD to find the destination(s). The significant point is not that System 2000, IMS, and TOTAL all have similar string catalogs when the data is structured similarly, but that the string catalog represents completely all the various types of access paths regardless of the logical data structure.

```
DBD       NAME=AIRLINE,ACCESS=HDAM,
DATASET   DD1=AIRLHDAM,DEVICE=3330,..

SEGM      NAME=AIRPLANE,BYTES=20,FREQ=1,000,PTR=H,PARENT=0
FIELD     NAME=PLANE_ID, ,BYTES=8,START=1,TYPE=C
FIELD     NAME=P_TYPE,BYTES=4mSTART=9mTYPE=C
FIELD     NAME=P_LOC,BYTES=3,START=11,TYPE=(C)
FIELD     NAME=P_DEST,BYTES=3,START=14,TYPE=(C)
FIELD     NAME=FLT_NUM,BYTES=3,START=17,TYPE=C

SEGM      NAME=PASSENGE,BYTES=     FREQ=50,PTR=H,PARENT=AIRPLAND
FIELD     NAME=PASSNAME,BYTES=12,START=1,TYPE=(C)
FIELD     NAME=P_SEAT,BYTES=2,START=13,TYPE=C
FIELD     NAME=P_ADDR,BYTES=15,START=15,TYPE=C
```

(a)

```
          PLANE_ID
          P_TYPE
          P_LOC
          P_DEST
          FLT NUM

          PASSNAME
          P_SEAT
          P_ADDR
```

(b)

Figure 14. Partial IMS DBD for plane passenger DB.

```
BEGIN MASTER DATA SET
DATA SET NAME=APLA
        .
        .
        .
APLA CTRL=8
APLA LKPA=8=PASS                /*L-STRING TO PASS FILE*/
APLA LKAI=8=AIRP
        .
        .
        .
END MASTER DATA SET

BEGIN VARIABLE ENTRY DATA SET
DATA SET NAME =AIRP
        .
        .
        .
AIRPLID=8=APLA CTRL                     KEY IDENTIFIER
APLALKAI=8=AIRPPLID                     LINK
AIRPTYPE=(4)
AIRPLOCA=8=LOCACTRL             /*KEYED IN LOCATION INDEX*/
LOCALKAI=8=AIRPLOCA
AIRPDEST=8=DESTCTRL             /*INDEXED BY DESTINATION*/
DESTLKAI=8=AIRPDEST
AIRPFLNU=(3)

        .
        .
        .
END VARIABLE DATA SET

BEGIN VARIABLE ENTRY DATA SET
DATA SET NMAE=PASS
        .
        .
        .
PASSNAME=8=APLACTRL             /*COMBINES PASSNAME & PLANE ID FIELDS*/
APLALKPA=8=PASSNAME
PASSSEAT=(4)
PASSADDR=(15)
        .
        .
        .
END VARIABLE DATA SET

(Not shown:  Master data sets for LOC & DEST indexes)
```

Figure 15. Total DML for plane passenger DB.

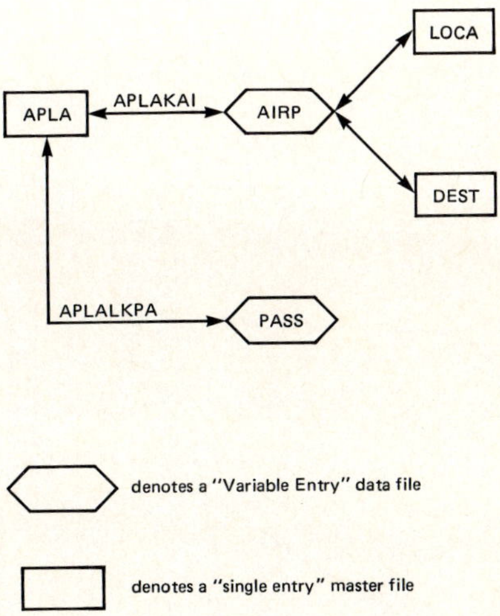


Figure 16. The file linkages in TOTAL for plane passenger DB.

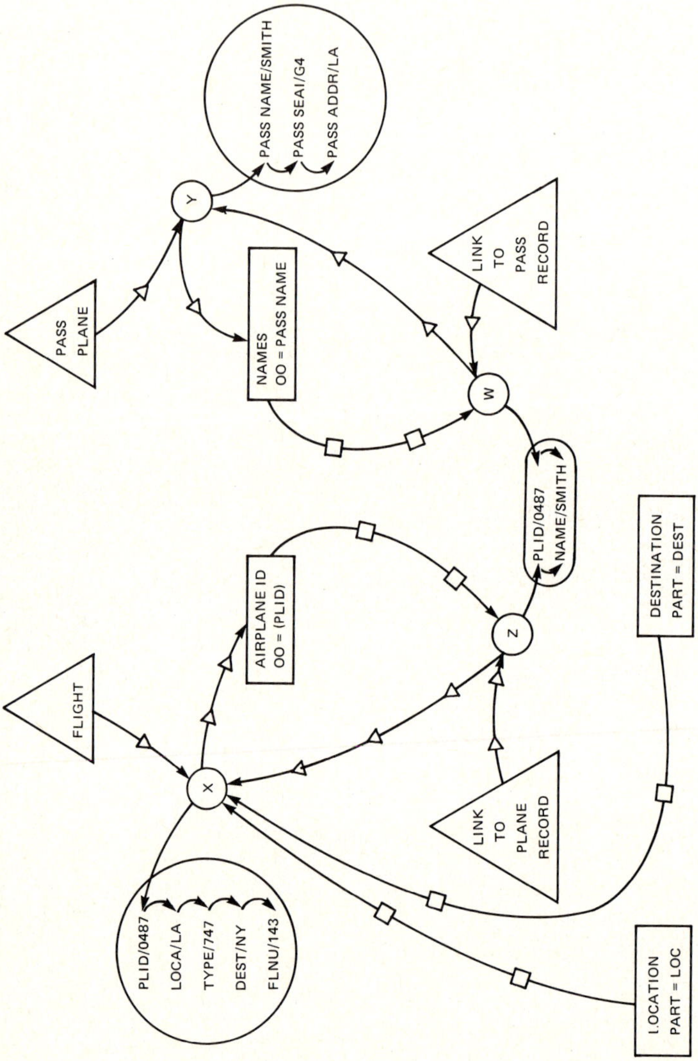


Figure 17. String model for the TOTAL plane passenger DB structure shown in Figure 16.

## VII. Conclusion and Summary

Our proposed approach to interconnecting heterogeneous DBMSs is to characterize the access paths into and through the data in a DIAM string catalog. Each DBMS will be responsible for maintaining a string table either locally or in some central directory. The string table of a DBMS will consist of a string catalog of the data at that DBMS and a table indicating how to traverse along each type of string, i.e., how that string is stored by the DBMS. A listing of which fields can be matched (i.e., PLANE # and PLANE ID) must be included. Optionally, some cost parameters may be associated with each string for optimizing string paths. If the string catalogs are not centralized, then a table of other nodes in the network must also be stored.

To answer a query, the string catalog is used to construct a string path to the desired fields and then the string table is used to actually retrieve (locate) those fields. This approach provides numerous advantages. Some of the main ones are (1) the indexing and access mechanisms of each DBMS is utilized as fully as possible; (2) the internal mechanisms of each DBMS are untouched so internal efficiency is not reduced; (3) each network user can use his own query language but host language level communication can also be supported. (4) no human interaction is required (for each query). If the cost parameters are included in the string table, then not only can the least expensive path be used but also, if several nodes must be examined, the search can begin with the least expensive.

We have developed and demonstrated through several examples a methodology for communication between different DBMSs. The technique is valid for different logical structures in different types of DBMSs on different computers. There are two parts to implement to provide a prototype: (1) a query-analyzer that inputs a query in a given language and a string catalog and produces a string path that "answers" the query in terms of the catalog, and (2) a string table for at least one DBMS.

Subjects of our future work include specifying the method for translating queries to string paths and the method for converting string paths into specific access requests on a given DBMS.

## ACKNOWLEDGEMENTS

The authors would like to thank Messrs Homer Yin and Howard Herron for their support of this work. They also would like to thank Ms. Barbara Wells for typing this report.

## VIII REFERENCES


1. A. Shoshani, "A Logical-Level Approach to Data Base Conversion," Proceedings, SIGMOD Conference, San Jose, California, 1975, P. 11.

2. B. Housel, D. Smith, N. Shu, V. Lum, "DEFINE: A Nonprocedural Data Description Language for Defining Information Easily" ACM Pacific Regional Symposium, April, 1975.

3. N. Shu, B. Housel, V. Lum, "Convert A High Level Translation Definition Language for Data Conversion", IBM Corporation, RJ 1500, San Jose, California, January, 1975.

4. N. Shu, V. Lum B. Housel, "An Approach to Data Migration in Computer Networks", IBM Corporation, RJ 1703, San Jose, California, January, 1976.

5. R. S. Marcus, "A Translating Computer Interactive for a Network Heterogeneous Interactive Information Retrieval Systems", SIGPLAN, January 1975.

6. M. E. Senko, E. B. Altman, M. M. Astrahan, and P. L. Fehder, "Data Structures and Accessing in Data Base Systems," IBM Systems Journal, Vol. 12, No. 1, 1973, P. 30.

7. M. M. Astrahan, E. B. Altman, P. L. Fehder, and M. E. Senko, "Concepts of a Data Independent Architectural Model", Proceedings of the ACM SIGFIDET Conference, Denver, Colorado (1972), P. 349.

8. E. B. Altman, M. M. Astrahan, P. L. Fehder, and M. E. Senko, "Specifications in a Data Independent Architectural Model", SIGFIDET Conference, Denver, Colorado (1972) P. 363

9. Wesley W. Chu and E. Nahouraii, "File Directory Design Considerations for Distributed Data Bases", Proceedings of the International Conference on Very Large Data Bases, Farmingham, Massachusetts, 1975.

10. System 2000 General Information Manual, MRI Systems Corporation, Austin TX 78766.

11. IMS/VS General Information Manual, IBM Publication No. GH20-1260, IBM Corporation, White Plains NY 10604.

12. TOTAL Reference Manual, Cincom Systems Corporation, Cincinnati OH 45211.

*Systems for Large Data Bases, P.C. Lockemann and E.J. Neuhold, (eds.)*
*North-Holland Publishing Company, 1976*

# APPLICATION PROGRAM CONVERSION DUE TO DATA BASE CHANGES*

Stanley Y. W. Su**
University of Florida
Gainesville, Florida

Advancement in hardware and software technologies and changes in the use environment of data base management systems often require that the data bases and their associated application programs be translated and converted in order to take advantage of newer technologies and new application needs. Research must be conducted to find efficient techniques for automatic or semi-automatic application program conversion, so that the expense and time involved in manual rewriting of application programs can be avoided.

This paper (1) describes the relation between data base translation and application program conversion, (2) identifies the program conversion tasks and their possible automation, (3) explores the techniques for solving the conversion problem through computer aided analysis of application programs, and (4) discusses and illustrates the data mapping operators useful for data base translation and their effects on program conversion. A semi-automatic approach to the conversion problem is proposed. It divides the conversion into two stages of analysis: data sublanguage statement analysis and conversion, and host language program analysis and conversion. Some conversion tasks and their analysis techniques are identified and described.

## I. INTRODUCTION

Advancement in hardware technology has facilitated rapid hardware turnover in an information system. Due to the lack of standardization in data structure and storage structure format, the data base of the system often has to be regenerated whenever machine and peripheral devices are changed. Also, a large data base is dynamic rather than static. New data are constantly entered into the data base while old data are deleted or modified. The use environment of an information system may also change. These changes are inevitable because of the natural growth of an institution. However, they may entail restructuring of the data base in many ways. First, the information structure of file represented by data model descriptions may have to be modified to account for the changes in data base semantics. Second, the data structures designed for data access purposes may have to be modified so that access to data can be carried out efficiently in response to users' new queries. Third, the physical structures may have to be changed to take advantage of the new hardware devices used.

Research on fully automatic data base translation has been undertaken by several research groups [8, 9, 15, 16, 18, 19, 20, 22, 23, 24, 25, 26, 29]. Our own re-

* This research is supported by NSF Grant MCS 76-100075.
** On sabbatical leave to the Department of Electrical Engineering, Taiwan National University, Taipei, Taiwan.

cent work [13, 27, 28] takes a semi-automatic approach to this problem by allowing an on-line user to browse, retrieve, edit, and restructure data files.

Another important and nontrivial problem, which is intimately related to the data translation problem, is the conversion of the set of application programs written for the old data bases. When a data base is converted into another one with a new data model description and a new logical and/or physical organization, the set of application programs needs to be modified to account for the changes in the data base. This is a very difficult process since the old programs, more often than not, are poorly documented and the programmers who wrote the programs might have already left the organizations. Consequently, either a set of new programs needs to be written or a group of programmers needs to dig painstakingly into old programs, attempting to understand what the original programmers were trying to do. This manual process is extremely time-consuming and expensive and is a waste of human energy. What we need, therefore, is a method of analyzing programs which will either do the program modification automatically or provide information to help the programmers do the necessary changes. Fundamental research needs to be conducted in this area to find a solution to this pressing problem facing the data processing community. This paper aims to analyze the problem and to identify the conversion tasks and possible approaches for solving the problem.

## II. SOME EXISTING WORKS

To this author's knowledge, there is no published material available on the specific subject of automatic program conversion. Nevertheless, several works have addressed themselves to problems related to it.

"Domain Migration," a topic well described by Codd [4], is a phenomenon where the data model definition (or schema in DBTG's terminology) is modified because of the changes in the relationships among the relations or because the relations in the data base are to be converted into the third normal form. Any change made in the data model definition will entail changes in the data-sublanguage statements used for manipulating and retrieving data in the model. This is true not only in relational data base systems but also in systems where other data models are used. Recent work by Codd [5] attempts to use a natural language as the query language so that it can be independent of the data model definition.

The work conducted in IBM San Jose Laboratory is significant. Lum, Housel, and Shu [11, 14] reported an interactive migration system, in which some problems dealing with program conversion due to application migration are discussed. At the present stage, the project emphasizes the development of a data translation aspect of the system, which uses a high level data description language DEFINE (Housel, et al. [12]) to define the source and target data bases. A high level language, CONVERT, (Shu et al. [21]) for data base mapping is also designed. Work on program conversion needs to be undertaken. In their study, the extraction of data structure, data usage and system information from application programs, and JCL or system tables (i.e., data base definition tables) are believed to be necessary for data base and program conversion.

Another work currently in progress is undertaken by Lewis T. Reinwald of the Bureau of Census [19] which attempts to convert procedural programs into a set of decision tables. The tables give a simple tabular representation of complex decision logic of the program. An algorithm which uses a push-down stack is developed for such conversion. Also, an algorithm for decomposing the decision tables into smaller ones is also available. This approach can be very useful for the program translation problem, since some kind of internal representation of complex program logic is a necessity for aiding the understanding of the programs.

In the context of code optimization in compilation, Ingalls [10] studied the execution profile of programs aiming to find the important part of each program where optimization of codes can bring great execution time efficiency. A program profile of an old application program can be very useful for writing an efficient new program.

From the limited works we can find, we see that the problem of application program conversion is not yet understood. How is data base translation related to the program conversion? What methodology can be taken to relieve the problem of converting programs manually? What information needs to be gathered from the application programs and from a data translation system regarding data base changes so that a program conversion system can carry out program conversion automatically or semi-automatically? How do data base changes affect the modification of the sublanguage and host language statements in application programs? All these and many other questions are awaiting answers.

## III. PROBLEM DEFINITION AND ANALYSIS

We shall define program conversion as a mechanism by which application programs for a data base can be modified to accommodate changes made in the data base and to meet the requirements in new applications. The program conversion problem can be divided into two broad areas:

(1) program conversion within an environment of a data base management system (DBMS),

(2) program conversion in an uncontrolled environment where programs and data bases are written and generated without the support of a data base management system.

### A. Within a DBMS Environment

In order to understand the problem within the first environment, the architecture of a data base system needs to be reviewed. The data base is a collection of interrelated data files containing the operational data of an enterprise. The data model [6] defines the files, their relations, and their mapping to the physical data base. It represents the logical view of the data base as seen by the data base administration. A data submodel is the interface which defines the information contents of the data base as it is viewed by a specific group of users, and specifies the mapping to the data model. A data sublanguage which can be embedded in a host language such as PL/1, COBOL, etc. is used by the user group to interact with the data submodel.

One of the goals of a DBMS is to achieve data independence. A change in the storage structure and access strategy should have no effect upon the user and his application programs since the data submodel is not affected by the change. However, if a data submodel is changed due to application migration, sublanguage statements for processing data defined by the submodel may have to be changed accordingly. Changes in sublanguage statements may in turn affect the host language statements and may require that the host program be modified. Therefore, the program conversion problem in the DBMS environment may involve two stages of conversion of the host language program.

The conversion of sublanguage queries involves the analysis of the queries and the modification of these queries to account for the changes made in the data model and/or data submodel. Whereas, the conversion of host language program involves the tracing of program logic, the identification of variable relations and program-subprogram structure, etc., the latter problem is a much more complex task.

### B. Within an Uncontrolled Environment

In an uncontrolled environment where data files are created, processed and accessed by individually written programs without the support of a DBMS (data model definition, data language and data processing facilities, etc.), the problem of program conversion correspondingly lacks structure. The scope of the problem is increased enormously by the great variance of programming styles and competencies of the application programmers. A poorly written application program will probably never lend itself to a systematic conversion process. In this environment, a program conversion system can at best aid the analyst in understanding the logic of the program and provide the information to identify the area of programs where changes need to be made. A semi-automatic system will be most suitable for performing interactive analysis of application programs.

We believe that the investigation of the automatic program conversion in the first environment will be more fruitful. However, it should be pointed out that the problem in the second environment is, in many ways, similar to the first one when a host language program is to be scanned and modified. The semi-automatic approach to be proposed for the conversion of a host language program can be used as an aid to solve the conversion problem in the uncontrolled environment.

The problem at hand is the conversion of the old application programs into a new set of programs suitable for the new converted data base. A system designed for achieving this task has at its disposal the following information:

(1) The structural description of the source data base.

(2) The structural description of the target base.

(3) The mapping from one structure to the other as described in some kind of mapping language, for example, in our semi-automatic system the retrieval and editing language (Su and Lam [27]) or the CONVERT language (Shu, et al. [21]).

(4) The set of application programs which were written for the source data base.

Based on these data, the system should analyze the application programs to determine what are the program statements that need to be modified given the information about the data base changes. It should be able either to make the program change automatically, or to identify the program areas or specific statements in which changes need to be made. The system also should be concerned about the efficiency of the modified programs and be able to accommodate those changes which the user wants to introduce and which are in addition to the modifications due to data base changes. If an application program is written in a host language such as PL/1 or COBOL which in turn calls a data sublanguage, conversion should be made on the sublanguage statements as well as those host language statements affected by the data base changes.

## IV. A GENERAL MODEL

The program conversion problem is intimately related to data base translation. A program conversion system would make use of the information regarding data base changes to make the corresponding program changes. Figure 1 shows a general model of program conversion as it is related to data base translation. In a data base translation system, a data definition language is used to define the source data base and the target data base. Some kind of data mapping language is used to specify the transformation from source data model to the target data model. Changes made in the data model often entail changes in the data submodels. Therefore the input to a program conversion system contains:

(1) the data model and submodel descriptions (schema and subschema in DBTG's terminology) of the source data base,

(2) the data model and submodel descriptions of the target data base, and

(3) the mapping (transformation) from the source to the target data base.

These data bases are used by a Data Migration Analyzer to construct a dictionary which contains all information regarding data base changes. When a user performs a data base translation which affects his data model and submodel, the data translation information (the data definitions and mappings) are analyzed by the Data Migration Analyzer which extracts the appropriate information and enters them into the Translation Dictionary. The changes in the migrating data base system is therefore continually documented.

The key component of the program conversion system is the Program Translator. The

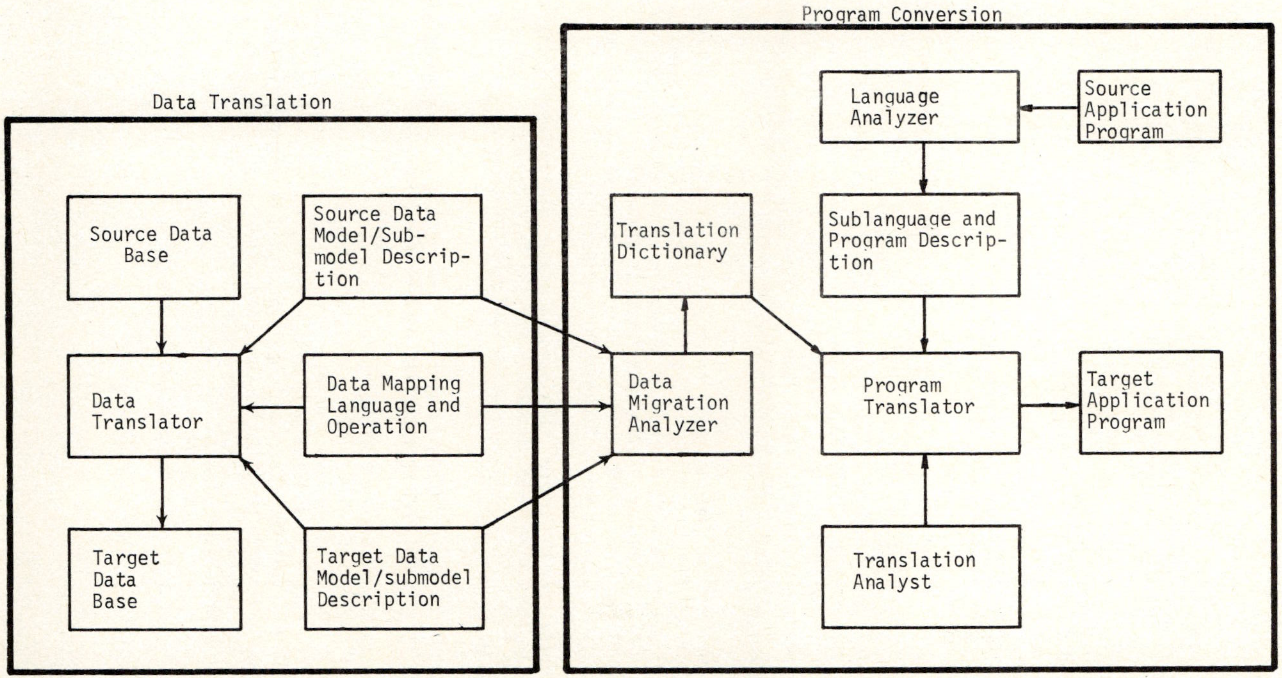


Figure 1. A General Model of Program Conversion as Related to Data Translation.

inputs to the Program Translator are the description of the source application program, the Translation Dictionary and the data provided by the interactive translation analyst. The Program Translator scans the source application program for data sublanguage queries. Once a query is encountered, the Program Translator retrieves information concerning the data changes which affects the data submodel used by the user. If possible, the Program Translator translates the query automatically. If not, the Program Translator interactively seeks help from the translation analyst and aids him/her in the construction of a new query.

If a new query can be constructed that is "equivalent" to the old query (either automatically or semi-automatically), this implies that the "identical" data (same variables and data types, but not necessarily the same values or same number of occurrences) will be available to the application program as before. In other words, the structure of the data submodel may have changed, but the data sublanguage query has been correspondingly changed so that the identical data are provided to the application program. In this case, any change in the data submodel is invisible to the host language program. Consequently, no change is needed for the host language statements and the translation process is completed for this query.

If an equivalent query cannot be constructed even with the help of the translation analyst, this implies that some data items that were referenced by the old query are no longer in existence. One possibility is that there was an error in the data translation process because a needed item has been lost through the data translation. If the deletion was not intentional, then some sort of recovery procedure must be initiated.

If the item was deleted intentionally and the associated application programs are intended to be modified accordingly, the Program Translator will provide information in helping the translation analyst in performing the second level of program conversion (i.e., conversion of the host language statements). It will help the translation analyst to understand the logic of the program, provide variable tracing, etc. (see conversion tasks described in Section V).

The Language Analyzer of Figure 1 analyzes an application program and produces a description of the sublanguage statements and the host program. The description can be in the form of data tables showing variable relations or decision tables representing program logic.

In order that we obtain a better intuitive or concrete grasp, examples are now presented to illustrate the concepts that were presented earlier.

For these examples, we assume the data conversion is accomplished by using the language DEFINE [12] and CONVERT [21], and that the data sublanguage SEQUEL [1] is embedded in the host language. We also assume that both the source and target data submodel are relational data models with the tables given in Figure 2. The DEFINE and CONVERT statements are presumably analyzed by the Data Migration Analyzer and the relevant information is extracted and stored in the Translation Dictionary. Now the Program Translator scans the source program and encounters the following queries expressed in the SEQUEL sublanguage.

Query 1: Get a list of departments (D#) which have a budget ≥ 100,000.

Source query: (Refer to Figure 2)

```
SELECT D#
FROM DEPT
WHERE BUDGT≥100000
```

Target query: (Refer to Figure 2)

```
SELECT DEPT#
FROM DEPTBUDG
WHERE BUDGET≥100000
```

This is an example of a simple query that is translated into another simple query. The Program Translator should recognize from the information that is stored in the Translation Dictionary that there is a one-to-one mapping for all the variables that are involved in the translation process (DEPT.D#-----> DEPTBUDG.DEPT# and DEPT.BUDGT----->DEPTBUDG.BUDGET). Only the variable names are changed. Therefore the structure of the query remains the same.

Query 2: Get a list of employees (E#) who work in department D#=101.

```
SELECT E#
FROM   DEPT
WHERE  D#=101
```

Target query:

```
SELECT E1#
FROM   PROJ1
WHERE  D1#=101
∪
SELECT E2#
FROM   PROJ2
WHERE  D2#=101
∪
SELECT E3#
FROM   PROJ3
WHERE  D3#=101
```

This is an example of a one-to-many mapping. The data items DEPT.D# and DEPT.E# of the source data submodel are now dispersed throughout three tables (PROJ1.D1#, PROJ2.D2#, PROJ3.D3#, PROJ1.E1#, etc.). The Program Translator recognizes and constructs a more complex but equivalent query to recover the identical data from the target submodel. In this case the required operation, a set union, is a result of the information that is stored in the Translation Dictionary.

Query 3: Get a list of employee names who work on PROJECT 2 and went to school at U of F.

Source query:

```
SELECT ENAME
FROM   DEPT
WHERE  E#=
       SELECT E#
       FROM   EMP
       WHERE  PROJ=2
       AND    SCHOOL='U OF F'
```

Target query:

```
SELECT ENAME2
FROM   PROJ2
WHERE  SCH2='U OF F'
```

This is an example of some <u>explicit</u> information in the source data submodel that has become some <u>implicit</u> information in the target data submodel. The data item, EMP.PROJ, of the source data submodel indicates explicitly the project membership of an employee. In the target data submodel the data item, PROJ, no longer exists.

SOURCE DATA SUBMODEL

DEPT

| D# | DNAME | DMGR | E# | ENAME | BUDGT |
|---|---|---|---|---|---|

EMP

| E# | SEX | PROJ | SCHOOL |
|---|---|---|---|

TARGET DATA SUBMODEL

PROJ1

| D1# | DNAME1 | DMGR1 | E1# | ENAME1 | SEX1 | SCH1 |
|---|---|---|---|---|---|---|

PROJ2

| D2# | DNAME2 | DMGR2 | E2# | ENAME2 | SEX2 | SCH2 |
|---|---|---|---|---|---|---|

PROJ3

| D3# | DNAME3 | DMGR3 | E3# | ENAME3 | SEX3 | SCH3 |
|---|---|---|---|---|---|---|

DEPTBUDG

| DEPT# | DNAME | DMGR | BUDGET |
|---|---|---|---|

---

Sample DEFINE description for source file EMP and target file DEPTBUDG:

<u>SOURCE FILE DESCRIPTION (EMP)</u>:

```
     ITEM E#:
        CHAR(PICTURE IS '9(4)');
     END E#
     ITEM SEX:
          :
     END SEX;
     ITEM PROJ:
          :
     END PROJ;
     ITEM SCHOOL:
          :
     END SCHOOL;
END FILE DESCRIPTION;
```

<u>TARGET FILE DESCRIPTION(DEPTBUDG)</u>:

```
     ITEM DEPT#:
          :
     END DEPT#;
     ITEM DNAME:
          :
     END DNAME;
     ITEM DMGR:
          :
     END DMGR;
     ITEM BUDGET:
          :
     END BUDGET;
END FILE DESCRIPTION;
```

---

CONVERT statements to create the target data submodel:

```
IEMP (D#,DNAME,DMGR,E#,ENAME,SEX,PROJ,SCHOOL) <----
     GRAFT  (EMP(E#,SEX,PROJ,SCHOOL) ONTO
             DEPT(D#,DNAME,DMGR,E#,ENAME):
             DEPT.E#=EMP.E#);

PROJ1 <----SELECT(D#,DNAME,DMGR,E#,ENAME,SEX,SCHOOL FROM IEMP:IEMP.PROJ=1)

PROJ2 <----SELECT(D#,DNAME,DMGR,E#,ENAME,SEX,SCHOOL FROM IEMP:IEMP.PROJ=2)

PROJ3 <----SELECT(D#,DNAME,DMGR,E#,ENAME,SEX,SCHOOL FROM IEMP:IEMP.PROJ=3)

DEPTBUDG <----DEPT(D#,DNAME,DMGR,BUDGT);
```

Figure 2. Data Model Description and Conversion

The project membership information is now implicitly indicated by the table in which the employee number is founded. Analyzing the DEFINE and CONVERT statements, the Data Migration Analyzer recognizes that the data item, EMP.PROJ, does not map into any data item in the target data submodel, but instead becomes implicit information. This information is stored in the Translation Dictionary which assists the Program Translation in the construction of the equivalent target query.

## V. CONVERSION TASKS

In this section, the tasks for the first stage analysis (sublanguage conversion) and the second stage analysis (host program conversion) are delineated. They represent the problems which need to be overcome before the implementation of a semi-automatic system can be undertaken.

### A. Tasks for the Conversion of Sublanguage Queries(first stage analysis)

#### 1. The Identification of Data Mapping Operators

One major area of our research is in the identification of the various ways in which source data items can be mapped into the target data items. Some of the mappings that have been identified are:

a. One source data item maps into one target data item--only the name is changed. (Example 1 of the previous section)

b. One item from one source table maps into more than one target table. (Example 2 of the previous section) In order to recover the data, a MERGE operation may be needed to be done to the target table.

c. More than one source data item maps into one target data item. A SELECT type of operation may be needed to be done to the target file to recover the data.

d. More than one source data item maps into more than one target data item. Then a combination of merging and selecting is necessary.

e. An explicit data item in the source data submodel maps into implicit information in the target data submodel. A SELECT type operation in the source query may provide the implicit information that is needed to recover the data. For example, as in Example 3 of the previous section, the implicit information indicates which table should be accessed in the target data submodel.

f. Implicit information in the source data submodel maps into an explicit data item in the target data submodel. The recovery would be similar to the reverse of (e).

g. Source file:
SALES

| ITEM ... FLOOR ... |
|---|

Target files:
SALES

| ITEM | ... DEPT# ... |
|---|---|

LOC

| FLOOR | ... | DEPT# ... |
|---|---|---|

Source query:

```
SELECT ITEM
FROM SALES
WHERE FLOOR='2'
```

Target query:

```
SELECT ITEM
FROM SALES
```

```
WHERE DEPT#=
      SELECT DEPT#
      FROM LOC
      WHERE FLOOR='2'
```

In the Translation Dictionary, it should be known that DEPT# is the common item used to tie together tables SALES and LOC in the target query. The primary key declared for each table gives this information.

h. Data recoding: In all of the mapping discussed before, the concern was the data item. In a data recoding mapping, the concern is the value of the data item. For example:

source data item ------ target data item

| SEX | SEX |
|---|---|
| 'MALE' | 0 |
| 'FEMALE' | 1 |

Of course, the recoding can be a great deal more complex and consequently attention is needed in developing a representation of such data recoding.

2. The Study on the Effect of Data Mapping Operators

The examples shown in the previous section examine the effect of a limited number of data mapping operators to the conversion of sublanguage statements. Many more data mapping operators such as the ones introduced in the CONVERT language and the editing language used in our own work on semi-automatic data translation have been studied. Another exemplification of the mapping facilities envisaged in the network data base organization is provided in the May, 1975, CODASYL JOD Subschema Mapping Functions [3]. These facilities provide multiple structures for record and set mapping a data base migration environment (e.g., MAPPING DIVISION, ALIAS SECTION, etc.). By working on examples using queries of different complexity and various mapping operators, we have gained insight into the data which should be gathered into the Translation Dictionary and the operations required for the Translator to make query modification. Algorithms for query conversion which account for the data base changes due to several of these data conversion operators have been obtained. A description of these algorithms will be considered inappropriate for this paper because they are quite lengthy and some are not yet completely evaluated.

A more general approach being investigated converts the data restructuring statements (for example, the CONVERT statements or others) and the source query into a common language, in this case an expanded relational algebraic language. Transformation rules are defined over the algebraic operators (Project, JOIN, Division, etc.) to restructure and modify the intermediate statement for the source query before translating the modified intermediate statement into the target query. This approach allows the target query to be formulated in a language different from the source language.

3. The Formalization of the Translation Dictionary

In our present work, the Translation Dictionary contains data tables which store general information about the reassignments of source relations and domains, the usage of target relations and domains, and the relations involved in the conversion operators. Data tables containing the specifics of each conversion operator are also established. These tables are established based on the input to the translation system described. They are used by the various algorithms for translating the source queries. Different algorithms are used for translating different general patterns of the source queries. Some examples of these patterns are:

simple SELECT-FROM-WHERE structure, nested structure, complex query structure containing optional intersection or union operators, and queries involving literal tuples. In our study, it has been clear that different language constructs require different transformation rules (or algorithms). An attempt is made to formalize the transformation rules and dictionary representations to allow a generalized program translator to be written which will handle the program translation task associated with different data base translation systems.

4. The Study of Translation Techniques

Investigation on the design and processing procedure of the Program Translator component are being undertaken to find the best techniques for scanning and modifying the sublanguage and host language statements, for processing and using the rules provided in the Translation Dictionary, and for interacting with the on-line user to provide him with help or to receive help from him to complete the translation task.

5. The Verification of the Correctness of Target Queries

The correctnes of a target query is dependent upon the correctness and the semantics-preserving properties of the transformation rules (or conversion algorithms). The rules selected for the program conversion rely on the data base conversion operators applied. The verification of the correctness of a target query is a difficult task. If the contents of the target data base has been changed by the data base conversion operators, we cannot judge the query's correctness by the data retrieved. In this case, we can only rely on the correctness of the transfromation rules or algorithms applied, or resort to the judgement of the interactive analyst. However, if the data base conversion involves only the restructuring of the data base (e.g., creating of new relations, splitting a large relation into several relations, etc.) and the renaming of relations and domains, it is possible to verify the correctness of a retrieval query by matching the data retrieved from the target data base with those retrieved from the source data base.

The approach being taken in our study is to reverse the involved content-preserving conversion operators to recreate the source data base and then to use the source query to retrieve data from it. The retrieved data should match the data retrieved by the target query, if the original data base and program conversion is correct.

B. Tasks for the Conversion of Host Language Program (second stage of analysis)

1. The Analysis of Program Logic

In order to perform program translation automatically or semi-automatically, the logic of the original application program must be made understood to the conversion system. This is because changes made in a data base may drastically affect the program logic required to access the data. Also modifications in one part of the program may affect the logic of the other parts. Thus, a clear description of the logical relations among the program statements needs to be generated and the logical flow of the entire program and subprogram structure will have to be produced.

In the analysis of program logic, there exists two levels of analysis: machine level and user level. In the machine level, there must exist an internal representation of the program logic such that it is accurate, complete, unambiguous, and is efficiently manipulated by a computer. In the user level, there must exist a high level representation so that a human user can act upon the program logic without being entangled in the details of the internal representation.

The mechanism that is under our prime consideration in studying the analysis of program logic is decision tables. The aspects of decision tables being studied are the following:

a. Program Instruction Block to Decision Table Transformation: The approach is to convert the logic to a tabular representation that can be manipulated easily and efficiently by a computer. Decision tables are suitable for representating complex logical structures of programs (Reinwald [19]). Effort is being made to develop methods to perform program-decision table transformation efficiently and, at the same time, for gathering other data from the programs.

b. Decision Table to User Interface: At the decision table level, it is extremely difficult, if not impossible, to manipulate the decision tables by a human analyst. The function of the interface is to allow the user to manipulate the decision tables using a high level language. The language is designed to allow the on-line user to extract information from the decision table and to make modifications on its contents. Study is being carried out to convert a decision table or portion of it to a flow-chart type of representation which is more readable to the user.

c. Decision Table to Program Instruction Transformation: Given a set of decision tables which were transformed from an instruction block and were modified by the user, methods are available to translate the tables into a set of instructions to carry out the logic represented by the tables. Works in this area have been thoroughly surveyed by Pooch [17].

### 2. The Analysis of Data Variable Relations

In program conversion it is important to determine how the data fields modified or deleted from the original data base are related to the other data variables in the programs. Take a simple example on data deletion. When a data field was deleted from the data records of a file, the program statements which read the data records have to be modified since the variable used for the data field in the statements needs to be removed. The removal of one variable may lead to the modification of the statements which use the variable. Also all other variables in a program which are a function of removed variable will have to be modified. The modifications may again cause chain reactions to other variables. Thus, the tracing of the interrelationships among the data variables of a program is necessary to facilitate program changes. Thus, the analysis of data variable relations is two-fold:

a. Analysis of the variables that are directly affected by the data translation.
b. Analysis of the variables that are indirectly affected by the data translation. Input to the program conversion system is the mapping of the source data to target data. From this mapping, the system is to have the capability of determining automatically the set of variables that are directly affected by the data translation. This set of variables can be displayed on-line for the user. Through an on-line editing facility, the instructions affected by any variable can be retrieved and displayed on-line. Using the Program Logic analysis portion of the system, the user can browse the program logic and decide what changes to the instructions are necessary.

   In addition to retrieving the affected instructions, another set of variables (from the instructions) are compiled. These variables are directly affected by the first set of affected variables. This operation can be extended to several levels until all affected variables have been identified.

### 3. The Recognition of Data Structure Changes

In the data base translation, the data structure of the target file may have been changed from the source data file. This structural change should be made known to the user so that correct access can be made by the new program. For example, an array structure in the source file might have been changed to a list structure in the target file. The portion of the program which accesses the array will have to be changed for accessing the list in which computation of the next list element or access through pointers is required. Again the information concerning this structural change can be extracted from the data mapping or conversion language statements that are part of the input to the program conversion system. The actual data conversion instructions that are related to the data structural changes can be retrieved and displayed on-line. Assuming the user is familiar with the data conversion language, he can see exactly what structural changes were made. A sample of the old data along with its converted counterpart can be displayed for further clarity.

An additional example of this type of dynamic translation of data structures is provided in the network model by the alternatives of the MODE IS CHAIN or POINTER-ARRAY implementation of set structures [2]. The implications of the latter alternative for rapid data restructuring require significant study before a feasible implementation could be undertaken.

### 4. The Recognition of Synonyms in Programs

Variable names used in a main program may be different from the ones used in a subprogram even though they refer to the same data. These variables are called synonyms. They can be defined by common blocks, external symbols, or by parameter passing. Recognition of these synonyms is important for tracing variable relations and program logic in programs and subprograms. Once the synonym relations among variables are identified, the problem on the identification of variable relations in the subprograms is the same as that of the main program. However, one precaution is that different calls to the same subprogram may require different changes to be made to the subprogram. For example, the paramenters which are passed to the subprogram in one call may be affected by the data file changes and thus require that the statements in the subprogram which use the arguments to be modified. Whereas, the paramenters which are passed on another call to the same subprogram may totally not be affected by the data changes. In this latter case, the statements in the subprogram should not be changed. Thus, modifications on subprograms need to take this problem into consideration. The program conversion system should allow the user to traverse from a subprogram to all places where calls are made to the subprogram. Interprogram structures and synonym relations will have to be gathered during application program analysis.

### 5. The Computation of the Execution Profile of Application Programs

The execution profile of a program is an instruction block vs time-in-execution "graph." The profile provides the work load of each instruction block. For example, if it is found from the profile that the program spends 85% of the execution time in a particular block of instructions, emphasis in efficiency should be placed mainly in this block of instructions during program conversion. Therefore, the execution profile of the old application programs can aid in the efficiency of the new programs. The program conversion system should analyze the old program and provide an execution profile of the old program. The user can be made aware of which parts of the program he should place the emphasis in order to produce a more efficient program.

## VI. SUMMARY AND CONCLUSION

The problem of application program conversion due to data base changes has been defined and analyzed. A model of program conversion and its relation to data base translation has been described. The program conversion process is divided into two stages of analysis: sublanguage conversion and host program conversion. Examples are given to illustrate how data sublanguage conversion can be carried out automatically. A semi-automatic approach is proposed to carry out the second stage of program analysis for host program conversion. The tasks relevant to both stages of analysis are identified and possible approaches to accomplish the tasks are proposed. It is this author's hope that the material presented will contribute to the future research in this important area.

What has been presented here represents the initial results of an ongoing investigation. The problem of automatic program conversion is far from solved. No conclusion can be drawn at this stage of research. However, based on our hand analysis of data mapping operators and application programs, we believe that the conversion of data sublanguage statements can be done automatically; whereas the conversion of host language programs should be carried out semi-automatically with the help of an interactive user. The problem of application program conversion is in a sense, dependent on the problem of data base conversion, which is itself an important yet unsolved problem. It is this author's belief, however, that both problems should be studied together because research work on the former problem can provide the necessary feedback to aid the formalization of the data base conversion rules and the formation of data mapping operators which are important in the total task of dealing with the data base migration.

REFERENCES

1. Chamberlin, D.D. and Boyce, R.F.,"SEQUEL: A Structured English Query Language," Proc. ACM-SIGMOD Workshop on Data Description, Access, and Control. Ann Arbor, Michigan, May 1-3, 1974.
2. CODASYL, Data Base Task Group Report, April, 1971, Sec. 3, p. 133.
3. CODASYL, Journal of Development, Data Base Facility, IV-4-1 ff, May, 1975.
4. Codd, E.F., "Further Normalization of the Data Base Relational Model," Courant Computer Science Symposia 6, Data Base Systems, New York, 1971, pp. 33-64.
5. Codd, E.F.,"Seven Steps to Rendezvous with the Casual User," Proc. IFIP TC-2 Working Conference on Data Base Management Systems, Cargese, Corsica, April 1-5, 1974, North-Holland, Amsterdam.
6. Data Base Task Group, "CODASYL Data Base Task Group Report," ACM, New York, 1971.
7. Date, C.J., An Introduction to Data Base Systems, Addison-Wesley, 1975.
8. Fry, J.P. and Sibley, E.J., "A Data Definition Language Approach to File Translation and File Conversion," University of Michigan, ISDOS Working Paper 44, 1971.
9. Fry, J.P., Frank, R.L., and Hershey III, E.A., "A Developmental Model for Data Translation," ACM SIGFIDET Workshop on Data Description and Access, 1972.
10. Ingalls, D., "The Execution Time Profile as a Programming Tool," in R. Rustin (ed.) Design and Optimization of Compilers, Prentice Hall, 1972, pp. 108-128.
11. Housel, B.C., Lum, V.Y., and Shu, N. C., "Architecture to an Interactive Migration System (AIMS)," Proc. of ACM SIDFIDET Workshop on Data Description and Control, 1974.
12. Housel, B.C., Smith,D.P., Shu, N.C., and Lum, V.Y., "DEFINE: A Nonprocedural Data Description Language for Defing Information Easily," ACM Pacific Regional Conference, San Francisco, 1975, pp. 62-70.
13. Lam, H. and Su, Stanley Y.W., "A Semi-Automatic Data Base Translation System," ACM Pacific Regional Conference, San Francisco, 1975, pp. 71-79.
14. Lum, V.Y.,Shu, N.C., and Housel, B.C., "Data Translation, PART I: A General Methodology for Data Conversion and Restructuring," IBM Research Report RJ 1525, July, 1975.
15. McGee, W.C.,"Informal Definitions for the Development of a Storage Structure Definition Language," ACM SIGFIDET Workshop on Data Description and Access, 1972.
16. Merten, A.G. and Fry, J.P., "A Data Description Language Approach to File Translation," Proceedings of the Workshop on Data Description, Access, and Control, 1974, pp. 191-205.
17. Pooch, V.W.,"Translation of Decision Tables," ACM's Computing Survey, Vol. 6, No. 2, June 1974, pp. 125-151.

18. Ramirez, J.A., Rin, N.A., and Prywes, N.S., "Automatic Generation of Data Conversion Program Using a Data Description Language," Proceedings of the ACM SIGFIDET Workshop on Data Description, Access, and Control, May 1974.
19. Reinwald, L.T., "The Re-Conversion Problem," a working paper, March 1974.
20. SDDTTG of the CODASYL Systems Committee, "Stored-Data Description and Data Translation: A Model and Language," working paper, 1975.
21. Shu, N.C., Housel,B.C.,and Lum, V.Y.,"CONVERT: A High Level Translation Definition Language for Data Conversion," IBM report RJ1515, Feb. 1975, to appear in the Communication of the ACM.
22. Sibley, E.H.,"Design Specification of a Prototype Data Translator," Progress report for ORA data translation project, Department of Industrial Engineering, University of Michigan, 1972.
23. Sibley, E.H. and Taylor, R.W., "A Data Definition and Mapping Language," Communication of the ACM, 16, 12, December 1973, pp. 750-759.
24. Sibley, E.H. and Merten, A. G.,"Transferability and Translation of Programs and Data," in Information Systems, COIN IV, edited by J.T.Tou, 1974, pp. 291-309.
25. Smith, D.C.P., "From a Data Description Point of View," Proceedings of the ACM's SIGPLAN and SIGIR Interface Meeting, November 1973.
26. Smith, D.C.P.,"A Method for Data Translation Using the Stored Data Definition and Translation TASK Group Languages," ACM SIGFIDET Workshop on Data Description and Access, 1972.
27. Su, Stanley Y.W., and Lam, Herman, "A Semi-Automatic Data Base Translation System for Achieving Data Sharing in a Network Environment," Proceedings of the ACM SIGFIDET Workshop on Data Description, Access, and Control, May 1974.
28. Su, Stanley Y.W., "A Semi-automatic Approach to Data Base Translation and Program Conversion," Proceedings of the International Computer Symposium, Vol. II, Taipei, Taiwan, 1975, pp. 172-180.
29. Taylor, R.W., "Generalized Data Base Management System Data Structures and Their Mapping to Physical Storage," Ph.D. Dissertation, University of Michigan, 1971.

*Systems for Large Data Bases, P.C. Lockemann and E.J. Neuhold, (eds.)*
*North-Holland Publishing Company, 1976*

# A DATA MANIPULATION LANGUAGE FOR RELATIONAL DATA STRUCTURES

J.H. ter Bekke
Eindhoven University of Technology
Department of Mathematics
Eindhoven
The Netherlands

Abstract

Some queries on a relational database are analyzed. This analysis results in new concepts for a high-level data manipulation language. In the proposed language the cardinal number concept from set theory is applied, using semantic information on the contents of a database. Each query formulation in this language consists of a small number of easily manageable expressions. This means that the simple relational data structures also are reflected in the programs which operate on these structures.

Keywords and Phrases: relational data model, data manipulation language, database, data structure, set theory, cardinal number, subset invariant.

CR Categories: 3.70, 4.22, 4.33, 4.34.

## 0. Introduction

A database consists of a collection related data, considered to be of interest for different applications. In the relational model [1], all data are represented in relations. Each relation contains data for a set of similar entities, such that every tuple in a relation represents one entity. In a relation the ordering of tuples is considered to be irrelevant. The same applies to the ordering of attributes which together form a relation.
With this datamodel mathematically inspired high-level data manipulation languages, e.g. based on the relational calculus and the relational algebra, were proposed as languages for databases [2,3]. Other languages were also developed which do not make use of these mathematical concepts [4].
These languages have a disadvantage in common, in that they often lead to one single and therefore formidable expression for a query on a database. In contrast with these languages, our proposal for a data manipulation language leads to a problem formulation which also for complex queries consists of a small number of simple expressions.
The key idea in this approach is the use of "subset invariants", which exist between database relations and which embody semantic information on the database. They naturally lead to the use of the cardinal number concept from set theory.

This paper consists of three sections. First a description is given of a sample database, which will be used in all examples. The second section gives an informal introduction to some concepts of our data manipulation language. The examples in this section have been selected to illustrate the retrieval part of the proposed language. Finally, a short comparison is presented with other data manipulation languages for relational databases.

## 1. Database definition

A relational database consists of a collection time-varying relations. Each relation in a database is used to represent data about a set of similar entities or data about a set of similar associations between entities. In the relational data model there is no difference between entities and associations.

The database definition provides information about the entity-types which are of interest to a community of users. For all applications it is the base of operation. A data manipulation language is used for maintenance and retrieval of data. The latter enables the user to select data from existing entities, but also to derive new information (possibly new entities) from them.

All examples in this paper concern a database which consists of seven normalized relations (i.e. attribute values are not compound values). In each relation one attribute or a number of attributes (called the primary key of a relation) uniquely identify the tuples; in the definition below these attributes are enclosed by square brackets.

<u>*rel*</u> *S*.[*sn*], *sname*, *location*

<u>*rel*</u> *P*.[*pn*], *pname*, *stock*, *min stock*, *max stock*

<u>*rel*</u> *A*.[*sn*,*pn*], *price*

<u>*rel*</u> *T*.[*sn*,*pn*,*date*], *quantity*

<u>*rel*</u> *C*.[*pn*,*dn*], *quantity*

<u>*rel*</u> *D*.[*dn*], *dname*, *location*

<u>*rel*</u> *E*.[*en*], *ename*, *location*, *dn*

<u>Semantics of these relations</u>

- Relation *S* contains data about suppliers. For each supplier are recorded the attributes: *sn* (supplier number), *sname* (supplier name) and *location* (city of operations).
- Relation *P* contains data about parts. For each part are recorded the attributes: *pn* (part number), *pname* (part name), *stock* (actual stock), *min stock* (lower stock limit) and *max stock* (upper stock limit).
- Relation *A* contains data about assortments, which are associations between suppliers and parts. This implies that the combination (*sn*,*pn*) appears as the primary key of the relation. Furthermore each association provides the *price* at which supplier *sn* can supply part *pn*.
- Relation *T* contains data about parts ordered. Each tuple in this relation can be considered as an association between a tuple from relation *A* and a *date* (date of order). Each association provides also the attribute *quantity* (quantity ordered).
- Relation *C* contains data about associations between parts and departments. Each association provides the *quantity* of part *pn* allocated to department *dn*.
- Relation *D* contains data about departments. For each department are recorded the attributes: *dn* (department number), *dname* (department name) and *location* (city in which it is located).
- Relation *E* contains data about employees. For each employee are recorded the attributes: *en* (employee number), *ename* (employee name), *location* (residence) and *dn* (department).

A database is not an arbitrary collection of entities. On the contrary, time-independent relationships exist between different sets of entities. In our database, the following relationship should remain invariant in time:
"The set of part numbers appearing in relation $C$ (denoted by $C^{pn}$) is a subset of the set of part numbers appearing in relation $P$ (denoted by $P^{pn}$)".
Mathematically: $C^{pn} \subseteq P^{pn}$.

Other invariants are: $A^{sn} \subseteq S^{sn}$ , $A^{pn} \subseteq P^{pn}$ , $T^{sn} \subseteq A^{sn}$ , $T^{pn} \subseteq A^{pn}$ , $E^{dn} \subseteq D^{dn}$ , $C^{dn} \subseteq D^{dn}$.
In what follows these invariants will more specifically be called "subset invariants". These subset invariants represent in fact consistency requirements, which the contents of a database must satisfy. An operation on a database could violate a subset invariant $X \subseteq Y$:

- when an element is inserted in the set *X*.
- when an element is removed from the set *Y*.

The maintenance of these subset invariants is considered to be a function for the database management system.

## 2. Selection from the database

In this section an informal introduction is given to the concepts which may be used in the formulation of queries on a relational database. These concepts will be introduced by examples. The following symbols are part of the definition language:

- braces: enclose optional parts of expressions.
- angle braces: enclose metasymbols.

### 2.1. The selection expression

The selection expression occupies a central position in our data manipulation language; it appears in each formulation of a query on a database. The general format of a selection expression will be:

*( <relation> { .<e list> } { | <predicate> } )*

Semantics: A selection expression will be used to obtain (usually new) tuples from a database. In this process only those tuples of *<relation>* must be considered which satisfy the *<predicate>*; in the absence of this *<predicate>* all tuples are to be considered. The expressions of the *<e list>* (i.e. expressions formed with at least one attribute of the relation) must be evaluated to yield the desired data in the new tuples. However, in the absence of *<e list>* all attributes of *<relation>* are provided. It should be noted that in a selection expression no elimination of duplicate (new) tuples is carried out (unless it is stated explicitly, see query 5). The *<relation>* { . *<e list>* } part of a selection expression is also called the "target", therefore *<relation>* will sometimes be called "target relation".

The next two simple queries illustrate the use of the selection expression. The first example is of the simplest form: selection of data using only one relation of the database.

Query 1. Get names of suppliers located in paris.

*get (S.sname | location = "paris")*

The verb *get* preceding a selection expression indicates that the tuples identified by the selection expression are to be output. From this formulation we see immediately that relation *S* must be considered; only values for attribute *sname* are to be output in this query. Moreover, because no projection is indicated duplicate values are not removed from this list.

We do not introduce the concept of a free variable in our manipulation language. That is why attributes in the target relation are indicated simply by their attribute name. For these attributes we will also use the term "primary attribute". Primary attributes in this example are *sname* and *location*.

In the next example we do not restrict ourselves to one relation of the database.

Query 2. Get names of employees who are not employed in their place of residence.

*get (E.ename | location ≠ D[dn].location)*

For each employee in relation *E*, we compare the value of the attribute *location* with the value of the attribute *location* in the corresponding tuple of relation *D*. The latter value can be found by using the value of attribute *dn*, which occurs in both relations. Because this attribute is the primary key of relation *D*, we use in our manipulation language the well-known notation of the subscripted variable.

An attribute that occurs in a relation associated with the target relation will be called "foreign attribute". The foreign attribute in this example is the attribute *D*[*dn*].*location*.

In the last example two (*location*) values from different relations are compared. This comparison can be performed because of the correspondence between the tuples from which the values are taken. This correspondence is provided by the attribute *dn*, which turns out to be the primary key in one of the relations considered. This kind of correspondence must always be present if attribute values of different relations have to be compared.
For the formulation of queries the restriction that only set elements can be referred to has no adverse consequences. On the contrary, it has a positive influence on the problem analysis (this is illustrated by example 5 of this section).

Henceforward we will distinguish the next four basic elements in a selection expression:

- Primary attribute: <*attribute*>
  A primary attribute is an attribute in the target relation.
- Membership test: <*relation*> [ <*key attribute*> ]
  The membership test *R*[*p*] is *true* if the tuple with key value equal to *p* occurs in relation *R*; otherwise it is *false*. This concept will be used in example 4.
- Foreign attribute: <*relation*> [ <*key attribute*> ] . <*attribute*>
  If the membership test part *R*[*p*] in the foreign attribute *R*[*p*].*q* is *true*, then *R*[*p*].*q* yields the attribute value *q* of the tuple in relation *R* with key value equal to *p*; otherwise it yields the value *nil*.
- Constants and variables of various types.

## 2.2. Use of subset invariants

Next to the primary key concept, the subset invariant is another important element in our formulation of queries. In all queries where otherwise sets would have to be compared, we aim at a description in which we can profit from a subset invariant. When using this approach, we are allowed to abstract ourselves from the actual contents of the sets; only cardinal numbers of sets (the number of elements in a set) are needed in the problem formulation. This approach is illustrated by the following examples.

Query 3. Get names of suppliers who are able to supply all parts.

The condition that has to be satisfied by the relevant suppliers is:

"All part numbers in relation *P* (denoted by $P^{pn}$) occur also in the set of part numbers *pn* in relation *A* that can be supplied by the supplier *sn* (denoted by $A^{pn}_{sn}$)".
Or in other words, does

$$A^{pn}_{sn} \supseteq P^{pn} \qquad (1)$$

hold.
Let $A_{sn}$ denote the subset of relation *A* corresponding with supplier *sn*.
From $A_{sn} \subseteq A$ and $A^{pn} \subseteq P^{pn}$ we have

$$A^{pn}_{sn} \subseteq P^{pn} \qquad (2)$$

Hence (1) can only hold if

$$A^{pn}_{sn} = P^{pn} \qquad (3)$$

Since $A^{pn}_{sn} \subseteq P^{pn}$ we may also equate the cardinal numbers:

$$count(A_{sn}^{pn}) = count(P^{pn}) \quad (4)$$

Since the combination $(sn,pn)$ is the primary key of relation $A$, any part number occurs at most once in a subset $A_{sn}$, so we may also investigate the following weaker condition:

$$count(A_{sn}) = count(P) \quad (5)$$

For each supplier in relation $S$ we need the cardinal number of the corresponding subset $A_{sn}$. For that purpose we could create a temporary relation $S'$ which, next to the attributes of relation $S$, also contains the cardinal numbers of the corresponding subsets in relation $A$. This is denoted by:

$$S' := S \oplus count(A_{sn})$$

Since relation $S'$ is obtained from relation $S$ by appending new information to entities in relation $S$, we will use the phrase: extending a database relation.

The notation introduced so far for the extension concept is not suitable to express more complex situations which can arise in queries. Instead we will use an expression similar to the selection expression. The general format of an extension statement is:

<u>ext</u> *<relation₁>* . *<attribute>* :

*<set function>* ( *<relation₂>* {.*<e list>* } <u>per</u> *<a list>* { | *<predicate>* } )

Semantics: An extension of *<relation₁>* with *<attribute>* is only defined if values for attributes in *<a list>* could occur as primary key values in *<relation₁>*. Then each tuple in *<relation₁>* corresponds with a (possibly empty) collection of tuples in *<relation₂>* which satisfy the *<predicate>*. From this collection of tuples another collection is obtained by selecting only those attributes that are defined in *<e list>*. The value for *<attribute>* in a tuple of *<relation₁>* is finally obtained by applying *<set function>* to the latter collection of tuples.
An extension of a relation is temporary, which means that it is only defined in the context of the query concerned.

The extension of relation $S$ with attribute *asm* using this concept would be:

<u>ext</u> *S.asm* : *count(A* <u>per</u> *sn)*

Relation $S$ may now temporarily be considered to read:

<u>rel</u> *S.[sn], sname, location, asm*

The following set functions may be applied on tuples in normalized relations:

*count*: delivers the number of elements in the corresponding collection.
*any* : delivers the value <u>true</u> if the corresponding collection is not empty, else the value <u>false</u>.
*empty*: delivers the value <u>true</u> if the corresponding collection is empty, else the value <u>false</u>.
*max* : selects the maximum of the expression *<e list>* in the corresponding collection; for an empty collection the value <u>nil</u> will be delivered. It is obvious that it can only be applied for attributes with a defined ordering.
*min* : selects the minimum value of the expression *<e list>* in the corresponding collection; for an empty collection the value <u>nil</u> will be delivered. It can only be applied for attributes with a defined ordering.
*total*: evaluates the sum of the expression *<e list>* of the corresponding collection; for an empty collection the value <u>nil</u> will be delivered. It is obvious that addition must be defined for the attributes in *<e list>*.

The following set function may also be applied on tuples in unnormalized relations (obtained from normalized relations):

*list*: selects the attribute values of *<e list>* attributes from the corresponding collection; for an empty collection the value <u>*nil*</u> will be delivered. The result is a compound attribute.

Next to an extension, we will need in the formulation of this query a variable which contains the cardinal number of a set. This can be realized by using the following assignment statement:

<u>*var*</u> *<variable> : <set function> ( <relation> { .<e list> } { | <predicate> } )*

Semantics: The result of this statement is that the value of the *<set function>*, applied to the selection expression, is assigned to a temporary *<variable>*. Excepting the function *list* all afore named functions may be used in this statement.

After these preparations the formulation of the third query now becomes self-explaining:

<u>*ext*</u> *S.asm: count(A* <u>*per*</u> *sn)*

<u>*var*</u> *p: count(P)*

<u>*get*</u> *(S.sname | asm = p)*

The execution order of the retrieval statements is by this formulation only partially fixed. Because the first two statements are independent of each other, they might be executed in parallel. However, the last statement is dependent on the results of other statements, therefore it must be executed last.

At this moment we can explain why set functions can not be used in the predicate or target of a selection expression. If a set function would occur in a selection expression, this would mean that the function must be evaluated over and over again for each tuple in the target relation. We can distinguish the following cases:

- The set function must be evaluated for each tuple in the target relation because the set function result is dependent on the values in the tuple. Before the selection of information can take place the creation of derived information is done separately by means of an extension. Within this creation process a temporary attribute is created which contains the set function result.
- The result of the set function is dependent on values in an associated relation of the database. In this case the associated relation should be extended with the desired attribute. The foreign attribute can be used to refer to this desired attribute.
- The set function provides a value which is constant for all tuples in the target relation. In this case it is obvious that a temporary variable should be created; the set function result will be assigned to this variable.

Using subset invariants, the formulation for the following query is rather obvious.

<u>Query 4</u>. Get names of suppliers who have at least the assortment of supplier s2.

The set of part numbers in the assortment of supplier *s2* (i.e. $A^{pn}_{s2}$) plays an important role in this query.
The condition that has to be satisfied by the relevant suppliers is:

$$A^{pn}_{sn} \supseteq A^{pn}_{s2} \qquad (6)$$

There is no subset invariant between these sets. Consequently, we may not use the cardinal numbers for verifying this condition; however, condition (6) is equivalent to the following condition:

$$(A^{pn}_{sn} \cap A^{pn}_{s2}) = A^{pn}_{s2} \tag{7}$$

A trivial subset invariant exists between the sets in this condition, so that we may use cardinal numbers:

$$count(A^{pn}_{sn} \cap A^{pn}_{s2}) = count(A_{s2}) \tag{8}$$

For the formulation of this query we will create a temporary relation. In our manipulation language this can be done by using the following statement:

*rel* <relation$_1$> . <a list> : ( <relation$_2$> . <e list> { | <predicate> } )

Semantics: By means of this statement a temporary <relation$_1$> is defined with attributes <a list> which are taken from <e list> of <relation$_2$>. In <a list> there must be at least one attribute enclosed by square brackets to denote the primary key of the new relation. On the right hand side of the colon a selection expression must be given.
(Note that whenever a key value occurs in more than one tuple as a result of the selection expression, then it is not determined which tuple will be included in the temporary relation.)

The formulation of this query is now:

```
rel R.[pn] : (A.pn | sn = "s2")
ext S.asm : count(A per sn | R[pn])
var asm s2 : count(R)
get (S.sname | asm = asm s2)
```

(Note: It is also possible to formulate this query without the creation of a temporary relation, namely by extension of relation $P$. The alternative formulation is left as an exercise for the reader.)

### 2.3. Derived entities

The foregoing queries were all straightforward, in the sense that attributes of existing entities were asked. In the next example we ask for attributes of entities that still have to be created since they are not present in the database.

Query 5. Get locations where at least three suppliers operate.

In this query we ask for locations of suppliers. Because there is no relation in the database with locations as entities, we must create such a temporary relation. This is done by a projection (denoted by [ and ]) of relation $S$ on the attribute *location*. Next, we must extend this temporary relation with the number of suppliers in each specific location. The locations for which this number is at least three, must be selected. Therefore, our solution to the problem will be:

```
rel L.[location] : (S.location)
ext L.count s : count(S per location)
get (L.location | count s ≥ 3)
```

### 2.4. Some simple queries

The following simple queries illustrate the use of other set functions.

Query 6. Get name and assortment for each supplier in paris.

```
rel R.[sn], sname : (S.sn, sname | location = "paris")
ext R.asm : list(A.pn per sn)
get (R.sname, asm)
```

Query 7. Get part numbers and names for unused parts.

*ext P.unused : empty(C per pn)*

*get (P.pn, pname | unused)*

Query 8. For each part get part number, name and total volume of parts on order.

*ext P.vol : total(T.quantity per pn)*

*get (P.pn, pname, vol)*

The following declaration can be very useful for the formulation of queries:

*def <relation>.<attribute> : <expression on attributes>*

Semantics: This form enables us to split up complex expressions on attributes into simpler expressions. The result of this declaration is the apparent extension of *<relation>* with *<attribute>*, the attribute value being equal to the evaluation of *<expression on attributes>*.

## 2.5. Stock control problem

We conclude this series of examples with a more complex problem which illustrates how a stock control problem can be formulated using the concepts of our data manipulation language.

The attribute *stock* in relation *P* denotes the actual stock of the parts. Parts for which the *stock* is below the minimum stock, must be ordered from one of the suppliers tendering the minimum price. The ordersize is equal to the difference between maximum stock and actual stock. Furthermore, a list must be given specifying for each order the supplier name, location and orderlines. The orders must also be added to relation *T* (the attribute *date* gets the value *"7603"*).
It is possible that a part to be ordered can not be supplied by any supplier. For these parts we want a list of part numbers and names.

We solve this problem by splitting it up into several simpler problems: We need the minimum price at which each part can be supplied. This is obtained by:

*ext P.min price : min(A.price per pn)*

Further, we have to know where the orders must be placed: A supplier is candidate to supply a certain part, if he is able to supply it at the minimum price for that part. Hence, a supplier number in an *A*-tuple is candidate if the price in the *A*-tuple is equal to the minimum price for that part in the corresponding *P*-tuple:

*def A.sn cand : price = P[pn].min price*

A part number in an *A*-tuple is candidate if the actual stock is below the minimum stock in the corresponding *P*-tuple, so we define:

*def A.pn cand : P[pn].stock < P[pn].min stock*

Next we define the ordersize:

*def A.supply : P[pn].max stock - P[pn].stock*

Now we can create a temporary relation *O* with all orderlines:

*rel O.[pn], sn, quantity : (A.pn, sn, supply | sn cand and pn cand)*

The insertion in relation *T* is obtained by the (herewith introduced) statement:

*ins T.sn, pn, date, quantity : (O.sn, pn, "7603", quantity)*

The list of orderlines is obtained by the following statements:

*ext S.orders : any(O per sn)*

*ext S.orderlines : list(O.pn, quantity per sn)*

*get (S.sname, location, orderlines | orders)*

Finally the list of undeliverable parts:

*ext P.no supplier : empty(A per pn)*

*get (P.pn, pname | no supplier and stock < min stock)*

This completes the formulation for this problem in our language.

## 3. Comparison with some other data manipulation languages

Rather than undertaking the formidable task of formulating the foregoing stock control problem with two other data manipulation languages for n-ary relational database systems, i.e. Alpha [2] and Sequel [4], we will present a nonexhaustive comparison of simpler queries. The Alpha language is a high level language based on the relational calculus; Sequel is based on so-called mappings.

The difference with these languages will be shown by some examples from the foregoing section. Firstly, we compare our language with Alpha:

Query. Get supplier names for suppliers who are able to supply all parts.

$$\{\ s.sname \mid s \in S \wedge \forall_{p\in P}\ \exists_{a\in A}\ (s.sn = a.sn \wedge a.pn = p.pn)\ \}$$

The relational calculus description is equivalent with the verification of the condition

$$A^{pn}_{sn} \supseteq P^{pn}$$

for each supplier *sn*, since in a relational calculus description subset invariants do not play any role. Hence, sets have to be compared instead of cardinal numbers of sets.
The single statement formulations of queries in the relational calculus leads, because of the nesting of quantifiers, to unmanageable expressions. (Even if the formulation could be split up into simpler expressions, we would obtain a description which differs completely from our proposal.)

The concept of primary key, which plays an important role in verifying the database consistency, is used heavily in our data manipulation language. On the other hand in Sequel no such concept exists. In the next example we see that such a concept facilitates a query formulation substantially.

Query. Get names of employees who are not employed in their place of residence.
In Sequel there are two possible (single statement) formulations for this query. Overlooking the primary key concept one might get a formulation analogous to Q 7 in reference [4].

```
select ename
from e in E
where dn in select dn
            from D
            where location ≠ e.location
```

For each employee we have to create a subset of department numbers (this subset may be pretty large). Furthermore, we must verify whether a given department number is included in this set.
This formulation may lead to a very time-consuming implementation. It is caused by the order in which the user has given the two "jointerms". This together with the overlooking of the primary key concept leads to the description above.
In our language the user must specify the order in which the jointerms have to be evaluated and lean heavily on the primary key concept.
In this example we see that a formulation using Sequel has a network structure. For simple queries this has no unpleasant consequences, but complex queries are almost unmanageable.

## 4. Conclusion

The relational datamodel is often associated with high-level data manipulation languages based on the relational calculus or relational algebra. In this paper it is indicated that these languages lead to unmanageable problem formulations. The use of semantic information about relations in the database and the possibility of introducing temporary relations or temporary extensions of existing relations leads to an approach in which this disadvantage does not exist. Each formulation in the proposed language follows naturally from the problem specification. It consists of a small number of simple statements; each statement representing a necessary step in the derivation of the desired result. These statements form a description which is easily adapted to variations in the problem specification.

## Acknowledgment

The author is indebted to professor R.J. Lunbeck and to F.J. Peters and F. Remmen for their valuable remarks during many fruitful discussions.

## References

1. Codd, E.F. A Relational Model of Data for Large Shared Data Banks. Comm. ACM 13, 6 (June 1970), 377-387.
2. Codd, E.F. A Data Base Sublanguage Founded on the Relational Calculus. Proc. 1971 ACM SIGFIDET Workshop, San Diego, Calif, Nov. 1971, 35-68.
3. Codd, E.F. Relational Completeness of Data Base Sublanguages, Courant Computer Science Symposia. Vol. 6: Data Base Systems, Prentice Hall, Englewood Cliffs, N.Y. 1971.
4. Astrahan, M.M., Chamberlin, D.D. Implementation of a Structured English Query Language, Comm. ACM 18, 10 (Oct. 1975), 580-588.

*Systems for Large Data Bases, P.C. Lockemann and E.J.Neuhold, (eds.)*
*North-Holand Publishing Company, 1976*

# USER EXTENSIONS TO THE PETERLEE RELATIONAL TEST VEHICLE

Peter Hitchcock
IBM UK Scientific Centre
Neville Road
Peterlee
County Durham United Kingdom

In the design of the PRTV system we stressed the importance of the easy writing of extensions to the language, ISBL. We give sufficient details of the ISBL language to provide a framework in which to discuss these extensions. They fall into two classes, those which can be thought of as relations, computed when required, rather than being explicitly stored, and those where a tuple in the result relation is, in general, formed from values taken from more than one tuple in the input relation. We discuss these extensions at a theoretical level, how they are defined and used, and how they are implemented. Finally we discuss the operation of 'glumping' or partitioning, in terms of relations not in first normal form. This provides a general way of looking at such operations as subtotalling.

## INTRODUCTION

At the IBM UK Scientific Centre, we have implemented an experimental database system called the Peterlee Relational Test Vehicle, or PRTV [8]. The language used is an algebraic one called ISBL, for Information System Base Language. This language is complete in the sense of Codd [5], but since this identifies only the basic capability that a relational system should have, we stressed the importance of the easy writing of extensions to the language.

We classify these extensions into two types. The first type of extensions comprises those which can be thought of as relations which are computed when required, rather than being explicitly stored. This would enable one to use computed predicates for selection, or to extend a relation by forming tuples with an extra component computed from the others, and still to remain within the relational framework.

The second type of extensions comprises those which cannot be represented by relations in first normal form. When they are applied, a tuple in the result relation will in general be formed from values taken from more than one tuple in the input relation. Examples of such extensions are functions which total or count objects in a particular column of a relation.

We also need to extend the concept of relations to include those which are not in first normal form, that is to allow relations themselves to be elements in tuples. This can provide a grouping operation which has been called 'glumping' elsewhere, [9]. Glumping is necessary to provide a framework in which to discuss such operations as subtotalling a column of a relation on equal values in other columns.

We will discuss these extensions at several levels: from a theoretical standpoint, how they are defined and used in the PRTV system, and how they are implemented.

Common extensions of the types described above are usually supplied built into a system; however such sets of system provided functions cannot be complete. We seek to provide a clean framework within which a user can easily define and use his own extensions.

## THE ISBL LANGUAGE

We present here only those parts of the current ISBL language which are relevant to this paper. For a more detailed description the reader is referred to [8].

### Definitions:

The basic atomic unit is an *object*. Objects are taken from distinct sets called *domains*. Information connecting objects is held in *relations*. A relation may be represented as a table, each row of the table being a *tuple*. All objects in each column come from the same domain, and each column is identified by a *selector* which is unique within a relation. The set of selector-domain pairs is the *type* of a relation or a tuple. A *relation* is a set of tuples of the same type. The order of tuples is not defined, nor is the column order. There are thus many possible tabular representations of the same relation.

A relation is in *first normal form* if it has the property that none of its domains has objects which are themselves sets. An *unnormalized* relation is one which is not in first normal form, (Codd [4]).

### Operations:

In the relational algebra the operators act on relations to produce new relations as a result. We make use of six operations - union, intersection, difference, selection, projection and join.

The three operations *union*, *intersection* , and *difference* have their normal set definition. For each operation the types of the input relations must be identical, and this is the type of the result. The operator symbols we use are '+', '.' and '-' respectively.

Selection produces a subset of a relation all of whose tuples satisfy some criterion. This criterion is called a filter and can be any boolean expression involving comparisons between objects from different components of a tuple, or between objects from the tuple and constants. The operator is ';'.

From each tuple in the input relation, projection produces a tuple with only those components present which have been named in the projection list, any duplicate tuples being purged. A second use of projection is to rename the selectors of a relation. The projection operator is '%' and '->' is used in the projection list for renaming selectors.

The operator join accepts two relations and performs an equijoin on those components whose selector names are common to both relations. It could be a full quadratic join if the sets of selector names are disjoint, or an intersection if both input relations are of the same type. The join operator is '*'.

Examples:

Current_loans:

| selector | name | book | loan | due |
|---|---|---|---|---|
| domain | name | acq_no | date | date |
| values | adams | 78912 | 751202 | 760102 |
| | jones | 52689 | 751118 | 751218 |
| | jones | 8154 | 751202 | 760102 |
| | wilson | 31655 | 750601 | 750701 |

Acquisitions:

| selector | book | name | title |
|---|---|---|---|
| domain | acq_no | name | title |
| values | 52689 | austen | northanger abbey |
| | 31655 | sewell | black beauty |
| | 8154 | pynchon | gravity's rainbow |
| | 78912 | lafarge | laughing boy |
| | 4259 | mcbain | fuzz |

Figure 1. Sample Relations

Dates have been encoded as yymmdd, and the date on which the loan was made, and the date on which the book is due back have been recorded. Acq_no is the domain of the aquisition numbers of books. The Acquisitions relation contains those books held by the library.

Using the sample relations given in figure 1, we give examples of the use of the operators.

1. Books borrowed by Jones which are overdue, where today's date is December 7th 1975.

```
List current_loans;(name = 'jones' & due < 751207)
```

2. Those people who have borrowed books.

```
List current_loans % name
```

3. The titles and authors of the books borrowed by Jones.

```
A = (current_loans ; (name = 'jones') ) % book
```

Relation A contains the acquisition numbers of books by Jones. We use the join operator to find the titles and authors.

```
List ( A * acquisitions ) % ( title, name )
```

4. An alternative solution to example 3, would be to join current_loans with acquisitions and then to project out the required information. It will then be necessary to change the selectors of the acquisitions relation to avoid answering the question - find the titles of books borrowed by their authors. The alternative solution is:

```
List (current_loans*(acquisitions%(book,title,name->author)) ;
     (name = 'jones') % (author,title)
```

## USER EXTENSIONS

We are now in a position to describe how extensions, which add computational power to the language outlined above, are defined and used. Our aim is to develop the concepts for these extensions within the relational framework, and then to develop a useable concrete syntax.

### Tuple oriented Extensions

The Theoretical Basis:

The theoretical underpinning for this class of extensions proceeds as follows. Imagine that we need to produce a relation which gives the names of borrowers whose books are overdue, and the length of time that these books have been overdue. We would do this in the following way:

Let date_difference be an infinite relation of degree 3, with selector names date1, date2 and number_of_days, which is defined by the characteristic function:
number_of_days = date2 - date1, where minus is suitably computed.
The required result is given by:

A = (current_loans;due<751207) % (name,due)

A contains the names and due dates of overdue books.

We now add a extra component to each tuple in A by performing a quadratic join of A to a literal tuple.

B = A * <:751207:date:today:>

The brackets <: and :> enclose a literal tuple with selector name today, whose content is taken from the domain date.

The components of B are renamed to agree with the appropriate selectors of the computed relation date_difference.

C = B % (due->date1, today->date2, name) * date_difference

The result C has selectors date1, date2, number_of_days and name. We then project out only those columns required for the result.

List C % (name, number_of_days)

Date_difference:

| date1 | date2 | number_of_days |
|---|---|---|
| date | date | n |
| ... | ... | ... |
| 751202 | 760102 | 31 |
| 751202 | 760103 | 32 |
| 751202 | 760104 | 33 |
| ... | ... | ... |

Figure 2. The Infinite Relation Date_difference

Date_difference is an infinite relation whose tuples are computed as required from the characteristic equation:

date_difference = date2 - date1

where '-' is defined by a user extension written in PL/I.

An extension of the type illustrated above can be thought of as a relation in first normal form, with the property that given a <u>single tuple</u> of the correct type, it is possible to say whether or not this tuple is in the relation.

Relations of this type were first introduced in [6], where they are discussed more fully.

An alternative view, which emphasizes the orientation towards tuples, is to think, not of a computed relation R which is joined to its arguments A to produce a result B, but of a function F which acts on a relation to produce a relation as a result. ie B = F(A). Such a function F is said to be join representable iff there is a function g from a tuple t of the type of A to a relation of the type of B such that:

$$F(A) = \cup \{ < g(t) > \mid t \in A \}$$

Relating this back to our original view, this means that we can find a relation R such that:

(R * A) % X = F(A).

where X is a projection list which may remove some components from the joined relations to match the type of B.

A subset of the join representable functions given above is the class of functions whose defining function g maps a tuple from A to the empty relation or to a singleton relation. This subset is called the class of tuple in, tuple out functions.

The Language:

When we extended the ISBL language to deal with this type of extension, a mixture of the relational and functional views appeared. It is interesting to discuss the reasons for this choice. The relational view of extensions is important because it introduces them in a conceptually clean way. In practice however, it is somewhat clumsy. Computed relations will usually be used in a wide variety of contexts meaning that the renaming of selectors will normally be necessary, and also that some implicit conversions between domains will be needed to ensure that types match correctly for the join to take place. We do not have this domain conversion facility, and to include it in a general fashion might be dangerous. The notion of effectiveness also rears its ugly head. Some expressions involving computed relations might not be effective. This is discussed in more detail in [6]. For these reasons, the expression that used date_difference in our earlier example is actually written in ISBL as:

```
list B * date_difference(due, today | n:number_of_days)
```

Date_difference is regarded as a function, which takes as input a description of the type of the result relation required, and produces as a result a relation D suitable for joining to B. In more detail, the position of the arguments before the '|' define a renaming and the following argument defines the type of the result, with the meaning that the column 'due' is to be suitably subtracted from the column 'today' to produce a new column with selector 'number_of_days' whose values are taken from the domain called 'n'. The resulting relation has selectors due, today and number_of_days and is then joined to B.

The actual procedure that calculates the difference in dates is an I/O free PL/I procedure written to a certain protocol, which is compiled and linked into the system. In actual use, the framework of this procedure is set up in advance and all that the user supplies is the PL/I text required for the body of the procedure. There is no explicit reference to the storage and access mechanisms of PRTV. References [8] and [10] describe how the system is able to use such a procedure in an efficient manner. More detailed instructions on how to write and use these extensions will be found in [11].

The Implementation:

We intend to extend our implementation of these ideas in the near future. It is rather clumsy to express arithmetic and string expressions using functions such as Mult, Add, Concat etc., or to insist that such expressions are written as PL/I code and compiled and linked separately. We think that it is worthwhile to provide a more conventional framework for handling the common arithmetic and string functions and to allow these to be programmed on-line (ie without compilation ). The general mechanism can then be reserved for those functions which require extra programming capability not provided on-line, or which are going to be used frequently and are worth compiling and storing away. As an example of the level and type of function which we think appropiate to provide on-line, consider that we have a relation R with selector names cost and tax_rate, and that we wish to form a virtual column called price. This could be done in the following way:

R # (price <- cost x (1 + tax_rate / 100))

Forgive for the moment the possible confusion caused by the dual use of '+'. The expression above can be seen as a way of specifying the computed relation between price, cost and tax_rate, on-line rather than off-line. This computed relation can then be thought of as being joined with R to produce the result relation. The new modification operator '#' takes a relation and a relation specification, called a selector expression, and produces a new relation. Using this notation, the previous example becomes:

List B # (n:number_of_days <- date_difference(due, today))

In our implementation the evaluation of a relational expression is deferred until its value must be computed. As each line is input it is incrementally compiled into a tree form, where each node is an operator and relations appear at the leaves of the tree. The importance of the tuple oriented user extensions is that they can appear as operator nodes in the evaluation tree and can then take part in the subsequent optimization before the tree is evaluated. We have implemented the class of functions earlier described as tuple-in, tuple-out. Further details can be found in [10].

## File Oriented Extensions

The Theoretical Basis:

Not all extensions are tuple oriented. To work out the average value of a particular column of a relation we need data from all the tuples to form the result. To enable extensions of this type to be written, we provide a general purpose relational file interface between a programming language and the database, in this case PL/I.

To access a relation from PL/I, one opens a relational file for reading. One of the parameters to this command is a relational expression. A snapshot is taken of the value of this relational expression and the contents are assigned to a relational file. Tuples are ordered in this file and it has a cursor. The cursor can be moved and the contents of individual tuples can be read by a PL/I procedure. In a similar way a relational write file can be used to transfer data from PL/I to the database. This is similar to the host language interface of DSL Alpha [3] and the Relational Data Interface of System R [1].

The Language:

The language used to access this relational file interface consists of a set of PL/I functions and subroutines. There are functions which return the properties of relations such as degree and cardinality, subroutines to open and close relational files, to read and write objects from a tuple, and to move the cursor through relational files. ISBL statements can also be invoked so that, for example, new relations and domains can be created. We would have preferred that the interface was oriented towards tuples rather than towards elementary objects; this was not possible because ISBL is an interpretive language, and PL/I is a language designed to be compiled. The natural data structure into which a tuple could be read is a PL/I structure, whose structures names are those of the selectors of the relation. To compile a PL/I program such structure names must be known in advance, whereas it is in the spirit of a query oriented relational system that relations are developed interactively and so their selector names are not known in advance.

A more detailed statement of the language will be found in [11].

The Implementation:

The implementation of this interface is straightforward. A tree form of the relational expression is built up as before, and evaluated as tuples are needed in the relational file. This means that very general functions can be written in PL/I to access and manipulate this data and to store it back as a modified relation. These functions can call each other, and the ISBL interpreter and are fully integrated into the system. However, such functions as the minimum or maximum value of a field in a relation could possibly be written more efficiently if they appeared as nodes in the evaluation tree having limited memory and taking advantage of implementation techniques not known to the general external interface. The problem is how to do this in general, without exposing unnecessary parts of the internal implementation.

## GLUMPING

Although it is possible to specify any operation on relations using the relational file interface, there is an important class of extensions which should be considered separately, and within the relational framework. These have the general structure: first partition the set of tuples into groups, and then act on each of the groups to produce one (or zero ) tuples which form a new relation. To return to our library example, we may want to find the number of books that each borrower has on loan. If we allow ourselves to think of relations whose components can themselves be relations, we can answer this question by the combination of two operations. The first is glumping, or partitioning of the relation into groups on equal borrower name; the second is the appplication of the cardinaliity function, COUNT, to each of these subgroups or subrelations. ( The word 'glumping', as far as we know, owes its origin to the Codasyl Information Algebra [9].)

Conceptually we could introduce glumping into our system by an extension of the rename operator, using the selector notation introduced in the Vienna Definition Language [7] to specify the structure. As an example, consider a relation R with selectors a,b,c. The expression R%(a,b->d.b,c-> d.c) restructures R into a relation of degree 2, with selector names a and d. The values of the second component are themselves relations with selector names b and c. The glumped relation R' is given by:

$$R' = \{ \langle a,S \rangle \mid \langle a,b,c \rangle \in R \longleftrightarrow \langle b,c \rangle \in S \}$$

ie we have partitioned on equal values of a. If we now extend the selector expression capability to include expressions on relations, rather than just selector variables, then our library example becomes:

```
A = current_loans % (name, book-> group.book)

List A # (name, number <- COUNT(group))
```

The separation of the two operations, that of glumping, and that of the application of the COUNT function can be clearly seen.

Current_loans:

| name | group |
|---|---|
| name | book / acq_no |
| adams | 78912 |
| jones | 52689<br>8154 |
| wilson | 31655 |

Figure 3. The glumped relation current_loans

---

The expression
current_loans%(name,book- > group.book)
has the three tuples shown above. Values in the group column are themselves relations with the selector name book.

---

The glumping operation extends easily to hierarchies of any level. The operation proceeds a level at a time, collecting components into subrelations, and then glumping these subrelations if the structure specifies it.

We must now consider the inverse operation of unglumping and the interaction of this and glumping with the other relational operations.

When a relation is glumped, it is given further structure, and has elements grouped together by equal values in other columns. A relation in this form is said to be <u>reduced</u>. Glumped relations behave exactly as normal relations with respect to the relational operations, although the resulting relations may not be reduced. Consider a relation A, with a tuple <a,{b,c}> , and a relation B, with a tuple <a,{b,d}> . The relation A ∪ B will have two tuples <a,{b,c}>, <a,{b,d}>. since {b,c}> and {b,d} are relations with different values, and so is not reduced. If the relation is now unglumped, we have the tuples <a,b>, <a,c> , <a,d> and it will be in reduced form on glumping again, ie containing only the tuple <a,{b,c,d}>. One further characteristic of the unglump operation is its behaviour with respect to the empty relation. The tuple <a,{ }> is a perfectly acceptable value for a glumped relation and might arise as the result of a selector expression, although it cannot arise as the result of a glumping operation. This tuple would disappear on unglumping. The properties of the glump and unglump operations would therefore include the following:

unglump(glump(R)) = R

glump(unglump(R)) $\neq$ R since
(i) R may not be reduced
(ii) R may contain the empty relation

glump(R $\cup$ S) $\neq$ glump(R) $\cup$ glump(S)
because of reduction.

In our work so far we have only considered glumping in a theoretical way, as a framework to provide a formal basis for such operations as SUBTOTAL. When we come to consider the implementaion, we can go one of two ways. We could allow the glumped relations described above to exist in their own right as a new type of relation which can be stored away permanently, or we can insist that the glumping operation is immediately followed by an operation which produces a conventional relation, and do not expose the intermediate glumped relation as a well defined data object. We favour the second approach: one of the attractions of relations is their simple structure, to allow the imposition of further structure could be a dangerous precedent. We would therefore provide a function call whereby the user would specify the grouping structure and the actual operation to be carried out. This is the approach adopted by the GROUP BY operator in SEQUEL [2]. However, this only permits a two level hierarchy. Should a more general operation be necessary, this can be specified through the relational file interface. Here a glumped relation will be presented as a partially sorted relational file, with tuples grouped together by like values on certain fields. If these repeated fields are not present we produce a simple hierarchy. This could be a useful presentation of a relational file for data entry and output. An important practical point is to design the interface, and the implementation in such a way that the functions such as TOTAL, MAX, AVERAGE etc., are specified only once, and can then be used both on relations, and also on the subrelations produced by glumping.

## SUMMARY

Relational systems provide a good method for the storage and retrieval of data but, in the main, lack the facility for performing and defining computations which are not already provided as builtin functions to the system. We have presented two types of user extensions to a relational system called PRTV. For the first type we considered the theoretical underpinning of computed relations and 'join representable' functions, the general PRTV extension mechanism for the extensions, and outlined how a subset of arithmetic and string functions might be handled online. For the second type PRTV allows access to the full range of PL/I statements via a special relational file interface. However, both for efficiency reasons and for convenience of specification, it is worthwhile giving special consideration to the operation of glumping, or partitioning. This can be handled either as the extension of conventional relations to include those which are not in first normal form, or by the provision of a specific additional operation. We favour the second view, but must await the reactions of users, as to whether the notion of simple hierarchies is appropriate for a relational system.

ACKNOWLEDGEMENTS

The new ideas presented here owe much to other members of the PRTV group at Peterlee. In particular the ideas for selector expressions came from Terry Rogers and Pat Hall; the definition of join representability and the modification operator are due to John Owlett and based on discussions with Stephen Todd; finally, the section on glumping was work done jointly with Pat Hall.

REFERENCES

[1] Astrahan, M.M. et al.:'System R: Relational Approach to Database Management', ACM Transations on Database Systems, Vol. 1, no. 2, June 1976, pp.97-137.

[2] Chamberlin,D.D.,Boyce,R.F.: 'SEQUEL: A structured English Query Facility', proc. ACM SIGFIDET Workshop, Ann Arbor, April 1974.

[3] Codd,E.F.:'A Data Base Sublanguage Founded on the Relational Calculus', Proc. 1971 ACM-SIGFIDET Workshop on Data Description, Access and Control, San Diego, California, November 1971.

[4] Codd,E.F.: 'Further Normalisation of the Database Relational Model', IBM Research Report RJ909, August 1971.

[5] Codd,E.F.: 'Relational Completeness of Data Base Sublanguages', in 'Courant Computer Science Symposia, Vol 6: Database Systems',ed. G.Forsythe, Prentice-Hall, 1971, pp65-98.

[6] Hall,P.A.V.,Hitchcock,P.,Todd,S.J.P.: 'An Algebra of Relations for Machine Computation', Proc. ACM Symposium on Principles of Programming Languages, Palo Alto, January 1975.

[7] Lucas,P.,Lauer,P.,Stigleitner,H.: 'Method and Notation for the Formal Definition of Programming Languages', IBM Lab., Vienna, Tech.Rep., TR25.087, June, 1968.

[8] Todd,S.J.P.: 'PRTV: A Technical Overview', IBM UK Scientific Centre Report UKSC0075, July 1975.

[9] CODASYL,:'An Information Algebra', Phase I Report - Language Structure Group of the CODASYL Development Committee, CACM, 5,4 (April 1962),pp190-204.

[10] Todd,S.J.P.:'Integrated Architecture for Transaction Specification and Optimisation in Relational Database Systems', IBM UK Scientific Centre Technical Note TN 38, June 1976.

[11] 'User Manual for the Peterlee Relational Test Vehicle', IBM UK Scientific Centre Technical Note TN 34, July 1975.

*Systems for Large Data Bases, P.C. Lockemann and E.J. Neuhold, (eds.)*
*North-Holland Publishing Company, 1976*

# A DEDUCTIVE CAPABILITY FOR DATA MANAGEMENT

Charles Kellogg, System Development Corporation, Santa Monica, Calif.
Philip Klahr, System Development Corporation, Santa Monica, Calif.
Larry Travis, University of Wisconsin, Madison, Wisconsin

This paper examines some of the problems and issues involved in designing a practical deductive inference processor to augment a data management system, as well as some of the benefits that can be expected from such an augmentation. A deductive processor design is presented that incorporates new techniques for selecting, from large collections of mostly irrelevant general assertions and specific facts, the small number needed for deriving an answer to a particular query.

## INTRODUCTION

In this paper we discuss some of the issues involved in adding a deductive capability to a data management system, and we describe a specific approach towards achieving this objective. Figure 1 illustrates the major components of our deductive data management system:

- A language processor that translates user input into a formal intermediate symbolism.
- A data management system* that retrieves specific facts (n-tuples of data values) from a data base as required.
- A deductive processor that uses general assertions (i.e., premises representing general rule-based knowledge about a data-base domain) to derive implicit information from collections of explicit data values.
- A control module that facilitates communication between the several components of the system and directs interaction between the deductive processor and the data management system during on-line question answering.

Listed below are some of the benefits to be expected from adding a deductive processor to a data management system:

- A deductive processor permits the extraction of information that is not explicitly stored but that can be inferred by combining specific facts in the data base with rule-based knowledge encoded in general assertions. This augmentation of the information-retrieval function can be especially important for very large data-base domains.

---

*In our prototype we use a relational data management system (see Codd (1970), Date (1975)). The research described in this paper is an outgrowth and extension of our earlier research on natural-language data management (see Kellogg et al. (1971), Travis et al. (1973)).

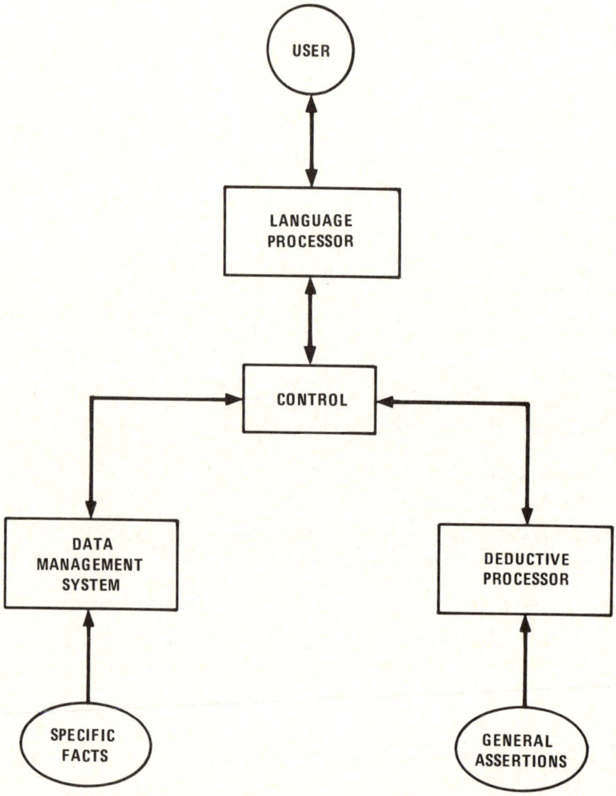


Figure 1. Deductively Augmented Data Management.

- A deductive processor allows a data management system's language to be extended and adapted to the needs of particular users. Thus a user's language can be uncoupled from the particular terms and categories used in organizing a data file. This is essential if users are to be able to use a system without having a thorough knowledge of its file structure. For example, a user should be able to ask whether the maternal grandfather of John Kennedy was richer than his paternal grandfather without knowing the respective men's names or that the file is structured in terms of net worth. Relatively powerful inferential mechanisms are necessary to enable full use of such descriptive references.

- A deductive processor not only generates answers to specific queries but also supplies evidence (lines of reasoning) for or against these answers. In some cases, the system may supply one argument leading to "yes" and another leading to "no" (indicating inconsistent information). In the real world of unreliable reports and uncertain facts, this kind of response will in many cases be much more useful to a user than simple categorical answers.

- While deduction is itself a precise and strict process, deductive arguments can use premises of differing degrees of plausibility. Since the plausibility of a conclusion (answer) is a function of the plausibility of the premises from which it is derived, deduction provides a basis for using "soft" information in a computer-based system. The important thing is that the system be able to show the user the evidence for a conclusion as well as the conclusion itself. Deduction can also be used to generate multiple distinct arguments for a conclusion, thereby supplying additional evidence for the plausibility of its answer.

- A deductive processor can, under certain circumstances, supply conditional answers when specific direct answers are not possible; e.g., "Is Joe Smith eligible for a pension?--Yes, if he has thirty years of continuous service." In this case the deductive processor identifies a specific fact about Joe Smith that it needs to complete an argument but that it cannot find in the files to which it has access.

- A deductive processor can answer "what-if" and other kinds of high-level queries that are difficult if not impossible for present-day data management systems.

Each of these capabilities is currently demonstrable within our prototype deductive data management system. Our primary concern in this paper is to outline our deductive system and to give examples emphasizing the derivation of implicit information.

Research on mechanizing deduction has been conducted primarily in the areas of question-answering and theorem proving within the broader area of artificial intelligence. Early question-answering systems such as SIR (Raphael (1964)), PROTOSYNTHEX (Schwarcz et al. (1970)), and CONVERSE (Kellogg (1968, 1971)) relied primarily on set-inclusion logic for their deductive capability. Elliott (1965) developed structure-specific procedures (such as one for transitivity and symmetry) for deriving new information from a file of specific facts. The inferential capabilities in these systems were limited and used for special purposes.

With the development of "resolution" (Robinson (1965)), more sophisticated theorem-proving techniques were incorporated into question-answering systems, most notably in Green (1969) and in Minker et al. (1973). General statements formulated in a first-order predicate-calculus symbolism could now be used to derive new information. Deductive power increased considerably, but at the expense of increased search space. This led to a host of resolution strategies (Chang and Lee (1973)). Some recent approaches to deduction have offered alternatives to resolution; these include procedure-oriented deductive systems, exemplified by PLANNER (Hewitt (1971)), and natural-deduction systems, exemplified by Bledsoe (1974) and Nevins (1974).

Our primary concern has been to design a deductive processor that will support practical data management in realistic environments involving large files of general and specific information.* We have concentrated on the problem of selecting from such large files the few premises and facts that are relevant for a particular required deduction. We have adopted some of the deductive techniques used in question-answering systems and modified them to be more suitable for data management; we have also introduced new "planning" techniques for premise selection. These techniques are discussed below.

## INFORMATION STRUCTURES TO SUPPORT DEDUCTIVE DATA MANAGEMENT

Figure 2 illustrates the principal files and processors that constitute our deductive system. Note that the deductive processor operates primarily on general assertions in its construction of proofs. The data management system accesses and retrieves specific facts when such facts are needed for proof completion. The four files used by the deductive processor are the general assertion file, the predicate connection graph, the variable substitution file, and the semantic advice file. These files have been segmented for purposes of processing efficiency and data organization.

General Assertion File. The deductive processor has access to a file of general assertions, or premises. These premises are represented in a Skolemized, quantifier-free form, as "primitive conditional" expressions. Primitive conditionals are logical statements whose major connective is the implication sign. On either side of this connective, groupings of literals may be combined conjunctively or disjunctively. Each literal is an atomic formula (i.e., a predicate and its arguments) or a negated atomic formula. The primitive conditional is a canonical form for the first-order predicate calculus. This form facilitates finding chains of deductively linked middle-term predicates, displaying inference plans and evidence chains, and storing information in such a way that the strategic or heuristic implications of the original formulation are not lost in the system, as is often the case with other canonical forms (e.g., the conjunctive normal form used in resolution).

A predicate occurrence is uniquely identified by specifying the premise in which it occurs, the predicate name of which it is an occurrence, its ordinal position in the premise, whether it is on the left or right of the main conditional, whether it is negated or not, and whether it is a member of a conjunctive or disjunctive set. For each predicate occurrence, the above information is represented by a unique compact bit string (a single IBM 370 computer word in our current implementation).

Predicate Connection Graph. The predicate connection graph is abstracted from the information available in the premises. Nodes represent predicate occurrences. Each edge between a pair of nodes represents a possible deductive interaction between the predicate occurrences in the nodes. The predicate connection graph is of key importance in our system. It represents explicitly and compactly a great deal of detailed structural information about general assertions and their possible interconnections. This information is in a form that can be quickly accessed and scanned.

---

*For the related artificial-intelligence problem of efficiently using a very large knowledge base, see McDermott (1975) and Fahlman (1975).

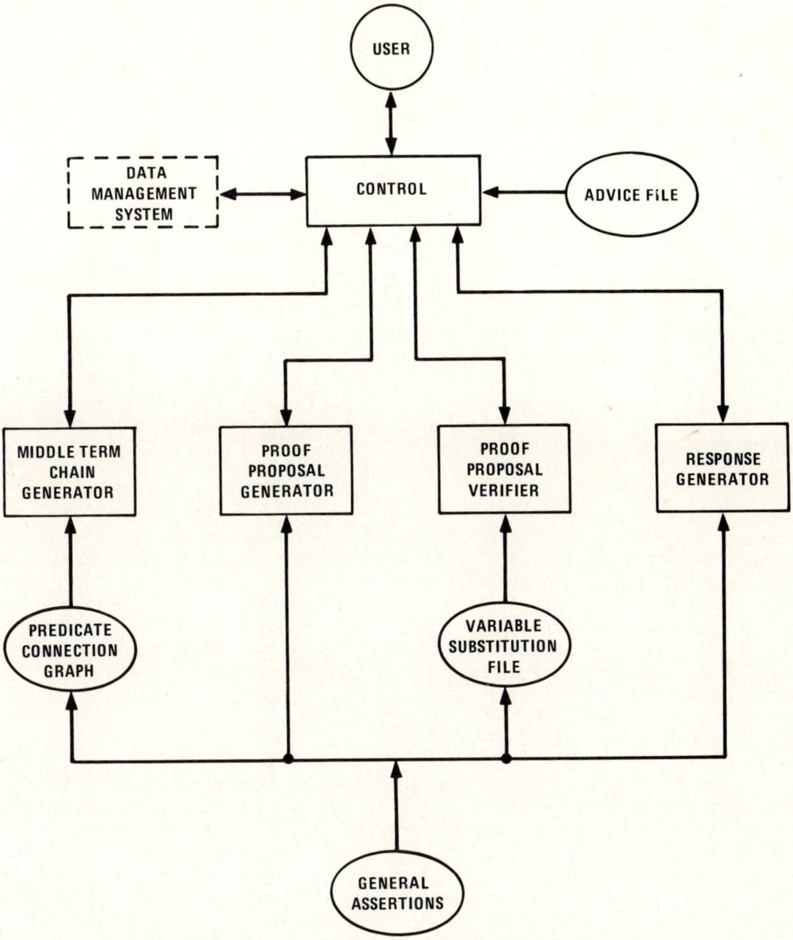


Figure 2. Deductive Data Management System Components.

The predicate connection graph bears some resemblance to the graph proof procedures of Kowalski (1975), Shostak (1976), and Yates et al. (1970). The important distinction between our approach and these procedures is in the way the connection graph is used. As we will see in the next section, the predicate connection graph is used to develop possible proof plans. The graph is an abstraction of information about premises and their deductive interactions and does not, by itself, construct proofs. It is used as a planning tool. For a full discussion of the predicate connection graph, its use in constructing proof plans, and the use of semantic advice in restricting searches through it, see Klahr (1975).

Figure 3 illustrates a small set of premises and their representations in primitive-conditional form. Figure 4 illustrates the predicate connection graph for these premises. The solid lines in Figure 4 are u-arcs (these "unification" arcs represent deductive interactions between different occurrences of the same predicate). These arcs are computed when premises are first entered into the system. Another kind of information in the predicate connection graph is the deductive dependency link, which represents deductive dependency between predicate occurrences within a single premise. Two of the four kinds of dependency links are shown in Figure 4.

Variable Substitution File. Another file, also separated out for purposes of efficiency, is the variable substitution file. This file is also abstracted from information in the premises. It consists of the substitutions for variables that establish the unifications represented by the u-arcs in the predicate connection graph. This file is used only during the verification process, when the substitution lists for all the unifications in a proof are combined and checked for consistency.

Semantic Advice File. Semantic advice can be of considerable aid in deductive searching. It permits the specification and use of deductively significant procedural semantic information specific to a particular domain of discourse. Frequently, advice cannot be formulated directly within the logical symbolism of the general assertions, even when a symbolism as rich as that of primitive conditionals is used. Whenever such advice can be captured, it can very likely be put to good use in simplifying and speeding up the deductive process. In the advice file, semantic advice is formulated and stored as condition-action pairs. (The user may also give problem-specific advice for any particular query.)

## DEDUCTIVE PROCESSOR MODULES

Control. The control module provides the primary interface between a user's symbolic input (queries, advice, and data), the several deductive processor modules, and the data management system. For example, Control may locate semantic advice in the advice file relevant to a specific input query. It may then call the Middle-Term Chain Generator and the Proof Proposal Generator to create proof proposals. Control will then invoke the Proof Proposal Verifier and the Data Management System in sequence to verify and complete a proof. Finally, it will call the Response Generator and display the answer and proof to the user.

Middle-Term Chain Generator. The predicate connection graph is used to find chains of middle-term predicates that deductively link the assumption and goal predicates of a query. The basic proof strategies of natural deduction, proof-by-contradiction, and proof-by-cases are automatically incorporated into this predicate chain generator (since the predicate dependency links reflected in the predicate connection graph are of the different kinds needed for all of these strategies; see Klahr (1975)). The chain-generation process may be visualized as one of generating a series of expanding "wave fronts" from each assumption and goal predicate. These wave fronts represent deductively significant possible paths from each predicate. As the two wave fronts expand, intersections are taken to determine when an assumption wave front impinges upon a goal wave front. When this happens, the system has discovered the beginning of a proof plan.

1. Husbands and wives are married to each other.

   $v(H(x_1,x_2), W(x_1,x_2)) \Rightarrow M(x_1,x_2)$

2. Marriage is a symmetric relation.

   $M(x_3,x_4) \Rightarrow M(x_4,x_3)$

3. Spouses of Greeks are Greek.

   $\&(G(x_5), M(x_5,x_6)) \Rightarrow G(x_6)$

4. People living in a place located in Greece are Greek.

   $\&(Loc(x_7,Greece), Liv(x_8,x_7)) \Rightarrow G(x_8)$

5. Spouses live in the same place.

   $\&(M(x_9,x_{10}), Liv(x_9,x_{11})) \Rightarrow Liv(x_{10},x_{11})$

Figure 3. Sample Premise Set in Primitive-Conditional Form.

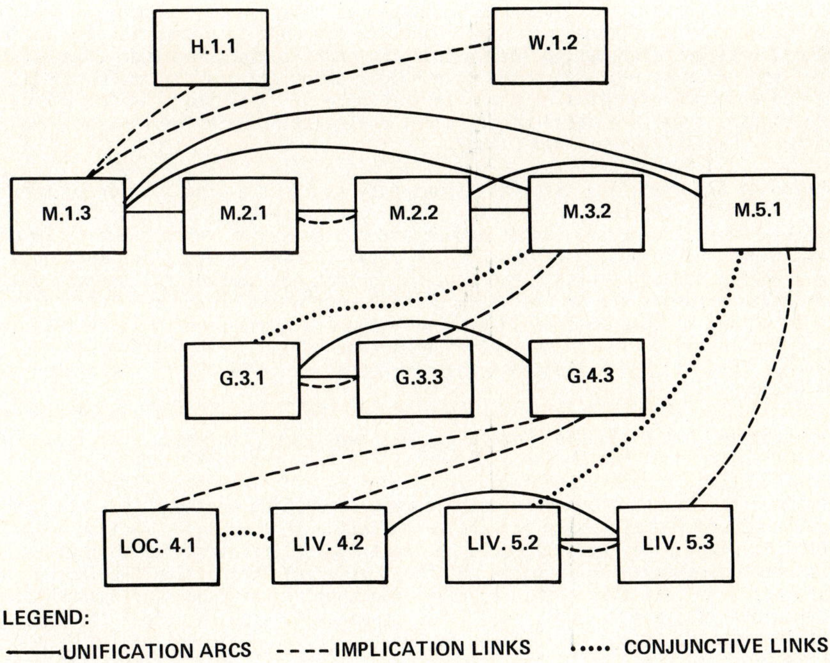


Figure 4. Predicate Connection Graph for the Sample Premise Set. (P.n.m is the occurrence of the predicate P in premise n, position m.)

Proof Proposal Generator. For each middle-term chain produced, the Proof Proposal Generator extracts the premises containing the predicate occurrences in the chain and forms skeletal proof plans. These plans are later sent to the verifier, which constructs full deductive detail for the proofs.

Proof Proposal Verifier. For each proof proposal, the variables and substitutions for them in the proof structure are examined to determine whether there are any blockages (variables taking on conflicting values). If verification is successful, the Control processor examines the proof to see whether there are any remaining subproblems that need support from the file of specific facts. If facts are needed, the data management system is called to search for these facts to complete the proof.

Response Generator. When the system completes a successful verification and instantiation of a proof proposal, it outputs answers and, if desired, the derivations on which they are based. When derivations are not complete, the system may display conditional answers or partial derivations that, in many cases, will provide clues to missing information that the user may be able to acquire from some other source.

## A BUSINESS INFORMATION EXAMPLE

As an example of how our system works, let us assume that we have the task of maintaining as complete and accurate a picture as possible of the operation of a large business organization. This will include the need to understand the various factions, real decision-making loci within the organization, and real flows of control and information, as opposed to publicly announced ones or the ones that appear on a formal organization chart as in Figure 5. This chart is for a fictional company that is a large distributing organization with three major line divisions: Chemical, Drug, and Liquor.

We should stress that high-level questions such as "Is the Drug faction or the Liquor faction in supremacy?" have to involve a considerable amount of human interpretation. A user should not expect a computer system, even one capable of sophisticated deduction, to generate categorical answers directly for such questions. What a deductive data management system can do, however, is help to collect and organize evidence for or against a general conclusion or working hypothesis. It is important to note that an inference system may make use of both certain and plausible information in the generation of arguments and in the display of evidence. That is, the evidence may be strong or weak; the human interpreter must judge which.

Let us suppose that a new man, Zembruski, has been appointed executive vice president and head of the Chemical division. We know something about him but this information is spotty and incomplete. The task is to work out deductive connections that might provide evidence toward concluding whether his appointment should be considered a victory for the Drug faction or the Liquor faction. For purposes of simplicity, we will focus on one principal relationship that might bear on this question. This is the notion of informal information flow among individuals. We take this notion to cover the possible exchanges of information between people who are friends, relatives, co-workers, spouses, etc. If we can obtain information that will allow us to deduce various instances of information flow, we might gain evidence, for example, that Zembruski has many more informational contacts with executives in the Liquor division than he does with those in the Drug division.

Suppose that Engler is vice president and head of Liquor. We can ask the question, "Will there be information flow between Engler and Zembruski?" Notice that while this is a yes/no question, we will not be satisfied with just a simple "yes" or "no." We will want to have access to the facts and the general assertions used by the inference mechanism in its derivation.

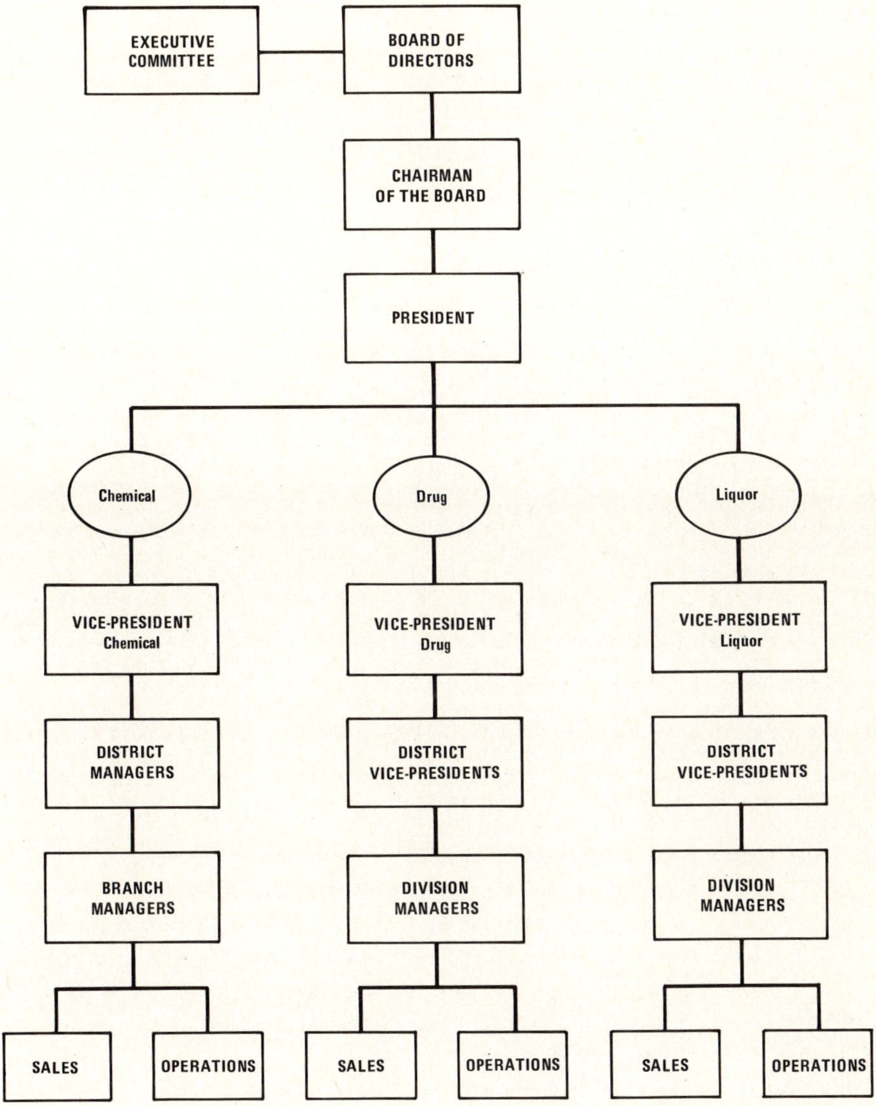


Figure 5. Organization Chart.

In Figures 6 and 7 we give an example set of specific facts and general assertions that are pertinent to questions of information flow. Of course, in an actual situation, there could be hundreds of additional general assertions in the system, and thousands of additional specific facts.

One successful derivation that our system could come up with, given the assertions and facts in Figures 6 and 7, is illustrated in Figure 8. When our system is given a complex question, it is broken down into a set of assumption predicates and a set of goal predicates. When both assumptions and goals exist, the Middle-Term Chain Generator is invoked to find middle-term predicate occurrences linking assumptions and goals. We will see an example of this process in the next example. For the current query we have only a single goal, namely, to establish information flow between Engler and Zembruski. In this situation the system will back up from the goal statement as illustrated in Figure 8 and select premises that can deductively lead to the establishment of the goal.

Each premise in Figure 8 represents an instance of a general assertion. The goal statement is enclosed in a rectangle, as are the two specific facts obtained from the data base. The vertical lines connecting the instances of predicates--for example, the line connecting two instances of Sibling--are unification arcs that are located by searching the predicate connection graph. It is within this graph that the system finds the linkages that enable it to link Brother to Sibling, Sibling to Relative, Relative to Nepotism, Nepotism to Friendship, and, finally, Friendship to Information-flow.

The general assertions used in Figure 8 are not all strictly true. For example, the premise concerning nepotism for relatives of subordinate employees is sometimes true (for certain circumscribed contexts or situations), but is clearly not always true. We anticipate many uses in our system of such plausible premises. Where this is done, it is clearly important to be able perspicuously to display to a user the lines of logical argument that are being followed by the system, so that the user can evaluate the credibility of a conclusion drawn from such questionable premises. Our system permits the discovery of alternative derivations for the same conclusion, which may enhance the credibility of the conclusion.

We note here a possible use of semantic advice. The user could suggest the use of particular premises or predicates that he feels may be appropriate to a particular query. For the current query, he may feel the premise concerning nepotism for relatives may be appropriate to establish information flow. The system would try

1. Zembruski is division head of Chemical: Head(Zembruski,Chemical)
2. Engler is division head of Liquor: Head(Engler,Liquor)
3. Richard Z. is a line subordinate of Engler: Line-sub(Richard Z.,Engler)
4. King is a line subordinate of Engler: Line-sub(King,Engler)
5. MR-Aces is a bridge club: Bridge-club(MR-Aces)
6. Rita S. is a member of MR-Aces: Member(Rita S.,MR-Aces)
7. Ann K. is a member of MR-Aces: Member(Ann K.,MR-Aces)
8. Rita S. is the wife of Smythe: Wife(Rita S.,Smythe)
9. Ann K. is the wife of King: Wife(Ann K.,King)
10. Richard Z. is the brother of Zembruski: Brother(Richard Z.,Zembruski)

Figure 6. Specific Facts.

1. Brothers and sisters are siblings.

   $\forall x,y$ ( v(Brother(x,y), Sister(x,y)) $\Rightarrow$ Sibling(x,y) )

2. Wives maintain information flow with their husbands.

   $\forall x,y$ ( Wife(x,y) $\Rightarrow$ Info-flow(x,y) )

3. Information flow runs between friends.

   $\forall x,y$ ( Friend(x,y) $\Rightarrow$ Info-flow(x,y) )

4. Every worker who is not a chairman of the board has a boss.

   $\forall x \exists y$ ( &(Worker(x), $\neg$ Chairman(x)) $\Rightarrow$ Boss(y,x) )

5. Every line subordinate is a worker and a subordinate.

   $\forall x,y$ ( Line-sub(x,y) $\Rightarrow$ &(Worker(x), Subord(x,y)) )

6. Every staff subordinate is a worker and a subordinate.

   $\forall x,y$ ( Staff-sub(x,y) $\Rightarrow$ &(Worker(x), Subord(x,y)) )

7. If someone does a nepotistic favor for another, then they are friends.

   $\forall x,y$ ( Nepot(x,y) $\Rightarrow$ Friend(x,y) )

8. Staff subordinates have information flow with their superiors.

   $\forall x,y$ ( Staff-sub(x,y) $\Rightarrow$ Info-flow(x,y) )

9. Line subordinates have information flow with their superiors.

   $\forall x,y$ ( Line-sub(x,y) $\Rightarrow$ Info-flow(x,y) )

10. There is a boss who has information flow with everyone of his subordinates.

    $\exists x \forall y$ ( &(Boss(x,y), Subord(y,x)) $\Rightarrow$ Info-flow(x,y) )

11. If someone is a subordinate of another, the superior may do a nepotistic favor for a relative of the subordinate.

    $\forall x,y,z$ ( &(Subord(x,y), Relative(x,z)) $\Rightarrow$ Nepot(y,z) )

12. People who are cousins or siblings are relatives.

    $\forall x,y$ ( v(Cousin(x,y), Sibling(x,y)) $\Rightarrow$ Relative(x,y) )

13. Members of a bridge club maintain information flow with each other.

    $\forall x,y,z$ ( &(Bridge-club(x), Member(y,x), Member(z,x)) $\Rightarrow$ Info-flow(y,z) )

14. The subordinate relation is transitive.

    $\forall x,y,z$ ( &(Subord(x,y), Subord(y,z)) $\Rightarrow$ Subord(x,z) )

15. Information flow is transitive.

    $\forall x,y,z$ ( &(Info-flow(x,y), Info-flow(y,z)) $\Rightarrow$ Info-flow(x,z) )

16. Information flow is symmetric.

    $\forall x,y$ ( Info-flow(x,y) $\Rightarrow$ Info-flow(y,x) )

Figure 7. General Assertions.

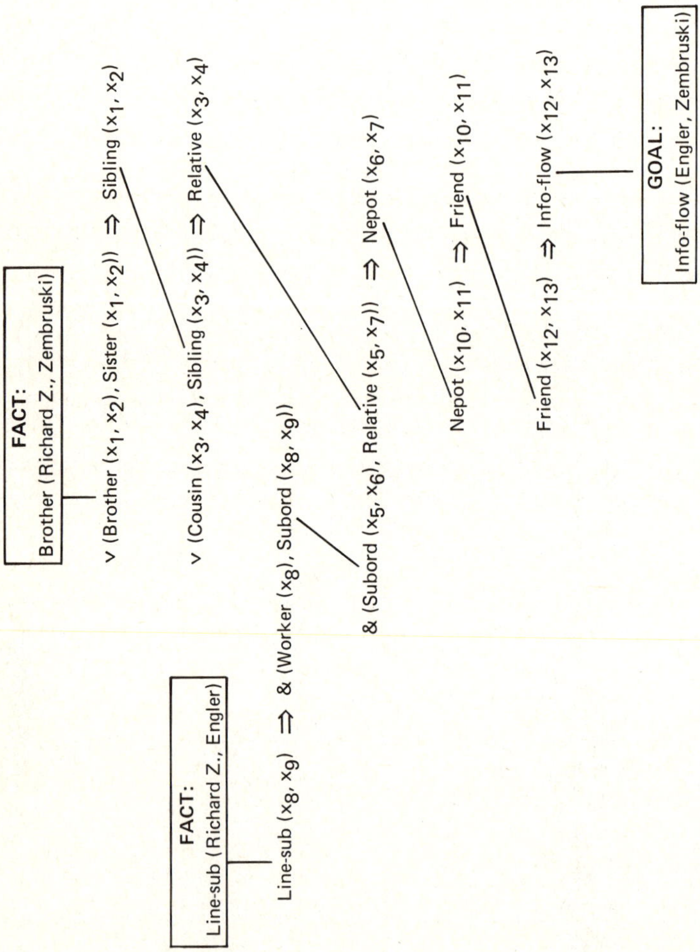


Figure 8. Derivation of Info-flow(Engler, Zembruski).

to use that premise in its proof. Similarly, if the user felt the relation "nepotism" is of key importance, the system would be alerted to link through occurrences of that predicate when possible. Note also that such advice could be placed in the advice file for general use (e.g., if goal is Info-flow, use Nepotism as middle term, or in more symbolic form "Goal(Info-flow); (Nepotism)").

To show another capability of the system, consider the following situation. We ask the system "What if Zembruski were to appoint Smythe to his staff; would there then be information flow between Engler and Zembruski?" Here we are suggesting the use of a particular assumption. Using this assumption the system will try to establish the same goal as in the earlier example.

A successful derivation for this query is shown in Figure 9. This proof uses premises quite different from those in the first derivation. This second derivation is more complex than the first. We can get the gist of the argument, however, if we follow through a few of the implications of the boxed specific facts that have been obtained from the data base. In order deductively to link Staff-sub(Smythe, Zembruski) to the goal Info-flow(Engler,Zembruski), the system has to determine that Smythe has a wife, Rita; that the MR-Aces is a bridge club; that Rita is a member of that bridge club; that Ann K. (the wife of employee King) belongs to the same bridge club, and hence, via a general assertion, has possible information flow with Rita; and that King is a line subordinate of Engler. Together, these relations deductively establish that there may indeed be information flow between Engler and Zembruski, namely through the wives of two of their subordinates.

We can use this example to show the basic operation of the system. The system is given an assumption and a goal. The Middle-Term Chain Generator attempts to find a chain of predicate occurrences that deductively link assumption to goal via the premises. The predicate connection graph, which contains information on the deductive connections between premises, is used in this chain-generation process. If the chain generator is successful and produces a chain, the Proof Proposal Generator extracts the set of premises containing the occurrences in the chain, and the system has the beginning of a proof plan. In Figure 9, the set of premises on the right were formed as a result of a chain linking the assumption to the goal via occurrences of the predicate Info-flow.

The Proof Proposal Generator then examines the set of premises to determine whether subproblems remain. In Figure 9, four subproblems were formed and are resolved using the four premises on the left. Subproblems resulting from these four premises are specified as needing fact-file support. (We have previously indicated to the system that certain predicates should be left for data-base search, either because we have complete knowledge about certain predicates such as Line-sub in an organization or because the information can be easily determined by the user, such as the wives of employees. In the latter case, the system would essentially be giving the user a "conditional answer," leaving certain subproblems open for user completion.)

Once all subproblems have been deductively resolved or left for fact-file support, the Proof Proposal Verifier combines the substitutions of all the unifications in the proof to check for consistency. Inconsistency occurs if a variable is required to take on two different constant values simultaneously. If verification is successful, the data management system is invoked to locate the specific facts needed for proof completion. In Figure 9, the six facts shown complete the proof.

While we have suggested the importance of displaying evidence for (or against) a deduced answer, we can readily see that derivations such as the one illustrated in Figure 9 may become difficult to follow. It is important to display machine-generated logical arguments in as perspicuous and user oriented a form as possible. We are currently developing techniques to display English-like formulations for such proofs.

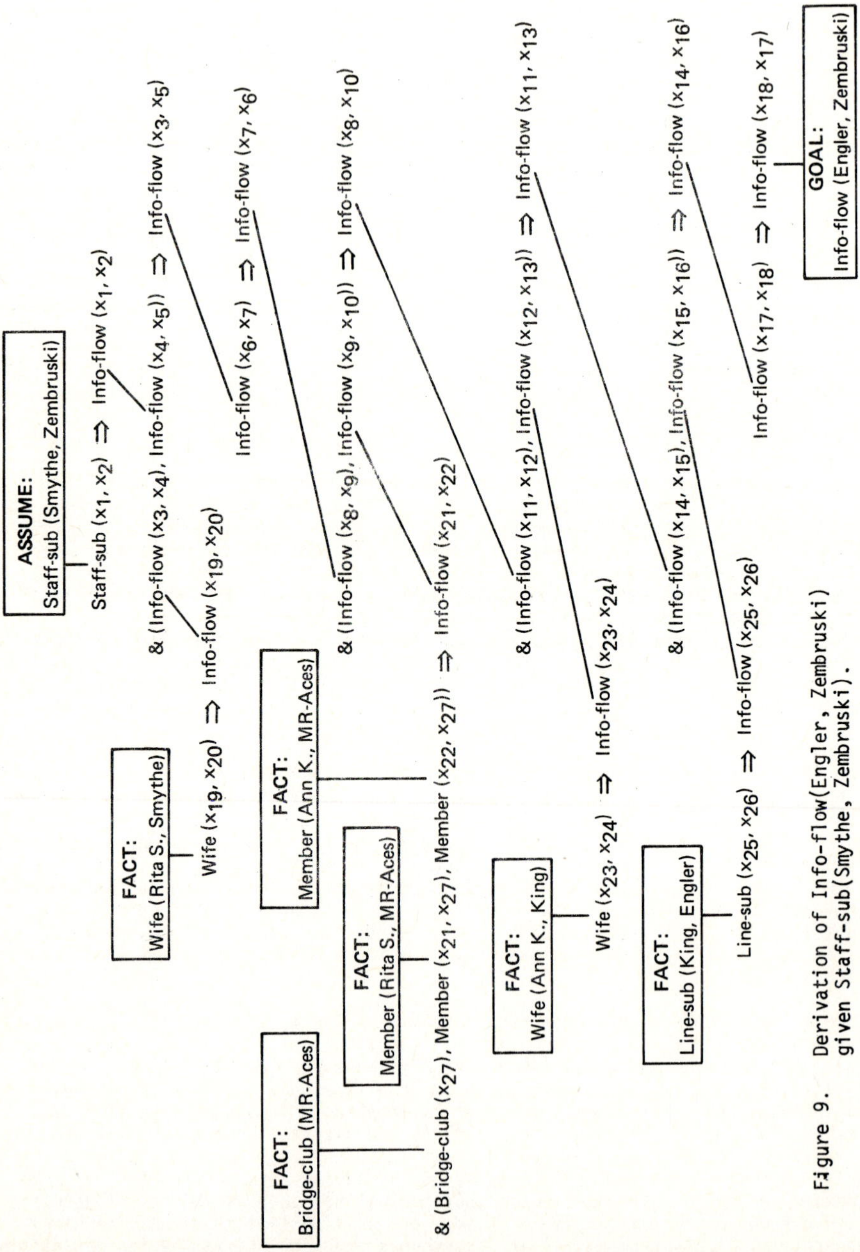


Figure 9. Derivation of Info-flow(Engler, Zembruski) given Staff-sub(Smythe, Zembruski).

## SUMMARY

We have argued that inference mechanisms can significantly enhance the power and usability of a data management system. They enable the compact storage of a large amount of information in the form of general assertions, and they enable the combination of these assertions, with explicitly stored specific facts, to deduce other specific facts that would otherwise not be available.

Perhaps just as important, a deductive capability in a data management system can enable extendability of user language. The general assertions used by the deductive mechanisms can definitionally connect the concepts used by the data management system for organizing its data base to different concepts more appropriate for a particular user community.

We have briefly described a deductive system specifically designed to provide inferential capability for a data management system. From various files containing information extracted from general assertions, the system generates middle-term chains, which it combines into proof proposals. These proposals are then used in the generation of data-base search requests for concrete facts, which, in turn, transform proposals into complete proofs and answers.

Applying deduction to practical question-answering in realistic environments requires special attention to the previously unsolved problem of efficiently selecting, from very large files of specific facts and general assertions, the very few that are relevant for a particular deduction. Our approach to this selection problem involves constructing abstract proof plans and then iteratively fleshing them out with more and more detail. Particular facts and assertions are selected for trial only when they fit into some plan. Semantic advice, i.e., advice specific to a particular subject domain, can be used to guide the construction and articulation of proof plans. On the basis of our experiments so far, the approach looks promising.

Acknowledgments: This work has been supported in part by the Advanced Research Projects Agency and System Development Corporation.

## REFERENCES

Bledsoe, W.W., and Bruell, P. (1974). A Man-Machine Theorem-Proving System. Artificial Intelligence, 5, No. 1, 51-72.

Chang, C.L., and Lee, R.C.T. (1973). Symbolic Logic and Mechanical Theorem Proving. Academic Press, New York.

Codd, E.F. (1970). A Relational Model of Data for Large Shared Data Banks. Comm. ACM, 13, No. 6, 377-387.

Date, C.J. (1975). An Introduction to Database Systems. Addison-Wesley, Reading, Mass.

Elliott, R.W. (1965). A Model for a Fact Retrieval System. TNN-42, Computation Center, U. of Texas, Austin.

Fahlman, S. (1975). A System for Representing and Using Real-World Knowledge. MIT AI Memo 331, Cambridge, Mass.

Green, C.C. (1969). Theorem Proving by Resolution as a Basis for Question-Answering Systems. In Machine Intelligence 4, Meltzer and Michie (Eds.), Edinburgh U. Press, Edinburgh, 183-205.

Hewitt, C. (1971). Procedural Embedding of Knowledge in PLANNER. Proc. Second Intl. Jt. Conf. Artificial Intelligence, British Computer Society, London, 167-184.

Kellogg, C.H. (1968). A Natural Language Compiler for On-line Data Management. Proc. FJCC, 33, Thompson Book Co., Washington, 473-493.

Kellogg, C.H., Burger, J., Diller, T., and Fogt, K. (1971). The CONVERSE Natural Language Data Management System: Current Status and Plans. Proc. Symp. Information Storage and Retrieval, U. of Maryland, College Park, 33-46.

Klahr, P. (1975). The Deductive Pathfinder: Creating Derivation Plans for Inferential Question-Answering. PH.D. Dissertation, Computer Sciences Dept., U. of Wisconsin, Madison.

Kowalski, R. (1975). A Proof Procedure Using Connection Graphs. JACM, 22, No. 4, 572-595.

McDermott, D.V. (1975). Very Large PLANNER-type Data Bases. MIT AI Memo 339, Cambridge.

Minker, J., Fishman, D.H., and McSkimin, J.R. (1973). The Q* Algorithm--A Search Strategy for a Deductive Question-Answering System. Artificial Intelligence, 4, No. 3/4, 225-243.

Nevins, A.J. (1974). A Human Oriented Logic for Automatic Theorem Proving. JACM, 21, No. 4, 606-621.

Raphael, B. (1964). A Computer Program Which "Understands." Proc. FJCC, 26, Spartan Press, Baltimore, 577-589.

Robinson, J.A. (1965). A Machine-Oriented Logic Based on the Resolution Principle. JACM, 12, No. 1, 23-41.

Schwarcz, R.M., Burger, J.F., and Simmons, R.F. (1970). A Deductive Question-Answerer for Natural Language Inference. Comm. ACM, 13, No. 3, 167-183.

Shostak, R.F. (1976). Refutation Graphs. Artificial Intelligence, 7, No. 1, 51-64.

Travis, L., Kellogg, C., and Klahr, P. (1973). Inferential Question-Answering: Extending CONVERSE. SP-3679, System Development Corporation, Santa Monica.

Yates, R.A., Raphael, B., and Hart, T.P. (1970). Resolution Graphs. Artificial Intelligence, 1, No. 4, 257-289.

*Systems for Large Data Bases, P.C. Lockemann and E.J. Neuhold, (eds.)*
*North-Holland Publishing Company, 1976*

# AN ENDUSER GUIDANCE COMPONENT FOR AN INTELLIGENT DATA BASE SYSTEM

R. Erbe
G. Walch

IBM Germany
Heidelberg Scientific Center
Tiergartenstr.15
D6900 Heidelberg

A general application guidance system -GAGS- was developed to offer a convenient enduser component for data base systems. It has the following four main features:

1. Dialogue supported methods dictionary: guides the user from a given application problem to the adequate solution method or program.
2. Dialogue supported data dictionary: gives syntactic and semantic information about the data available in data administration systems.
3. Dialogue supported execution facility: offers a system triggered execution of programs found with the help of the methods dictionary in order to process data identified by means of the data dictionary.
4. Dialogue supported system guidance: enables the unexperienced user to work with software systems without being a DP-professional.

The basic information structure for the interactive guidance which is the common basic concept of the four facilities listed above, is the information network. It is generated by breaking down the knowledge about the application area in question into information elements (network nodes) which are interconnected (network arcs).

## 1. INTRODUCTION

To enable the problem solver to make efficient use of software packages developed by computer manufacturers, software firms or computer science institutes, he should be offered a comprehensive and intelligible documentation. However, working with to day's conventional software documentation, most users, run into problems. The main shortcoming is the difficulty how to identify the suitable program for a given problem. This is due to the fact that there is insufficient guidance from a semantic point of view.

To overcome these difficulties, a General Application Guidance System -GAGS- is developed. In its function as a methods dictionary it guides the user from a defined problem to the respective solution method /2,3/. Methods are understood as implemented programs and abstract methods. This idea allows a guidance to a solution even if respective programs do not exist or if the problem is not tailored for a computerized solution.

Just as the system is used as a guide for program retrieval and use, it may also serve as a guide for data retrieval and use, delivering information about the data available in a system, e.g. their meaning, origin, use, format, and relationships, i. e. GAGS may function as a data dictionary.

Beyond the capabilities for information retrieval about programs and data, the system is extended to give interactive support for program execution by prompting the user for the specification of the arguments, and - optionally - by displaying explanations of the meaning of arguments and results. The specification may be done by value, by variable name, or by file name. In the latter case, the file description can be found in the data dictionary and used by system functions to access the data.

Finally, it should be pointed out, that the network concept described in chapter 2 allows to make the GAG-System selfexplanatory: it may contain as one of its applications the structured description of the GAGS usage, or of the usage of any other information retrieval and processing system, to which GAGS may be attached as a kind of man machine interface.

## 2. METHODS DICTIONARY

The interactive guidance system developed for the search and selection of problem solving methods is based on the following concepts:

The information about application areas and abstract methods including their prerequisites is separated from the conventional program documentation. It is broken down into small interconnected elements. The resulting structures may be understood as information networks /1,7/ with nodes representing information elements and connecting arcs leading from elements of general information to elements of more detailed information ( see figure 1 for an example ). Each node may have an arbitrary number of incoming and outgoing arcs.

The system offers elements of information in a systematic way such that the user is guided from more general to more specific information. In the most general case this implies a guidance from some application area via specific problems and subproblems to the adequate method and program.

The starting point for a method search depends on the user's knowledge. The user can begin at a node of general information or at a node of relatively specific information. In principle, every node is a possible entry node. If the user does not know what the content of the system is, he is offered a list of all application areas or problem fields for which documentation exists. But if he has general knowledge and wants some specific information he can directly identify the respective node.

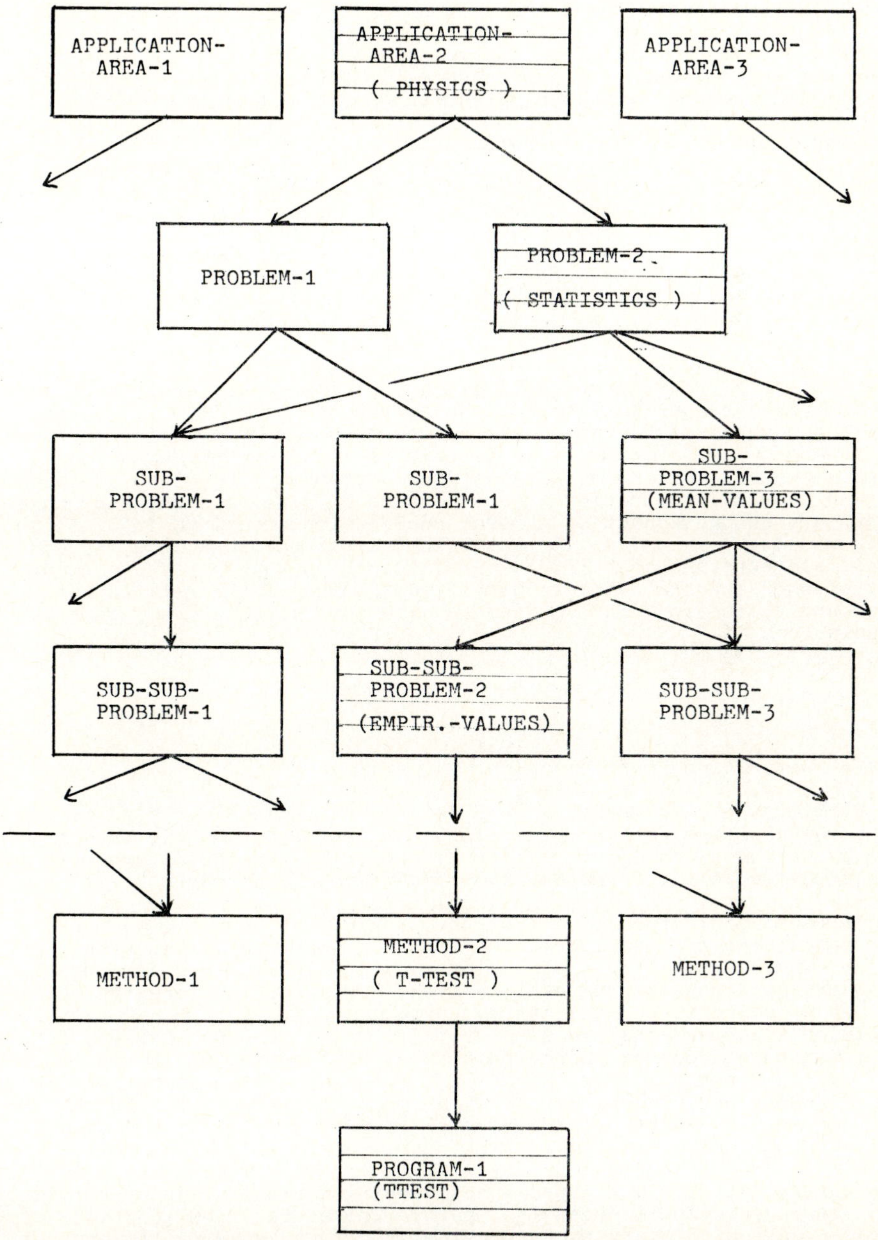


Fig. 1: Section of a General Method Oriented Information Network (one possible search path hatched, example from STATISTICS in parentheses).

Based on the information contained in this start node and in its immediate successor nodes the user has to decide to which of the successor nodes he wants to proceed . The selected successor becomes the current node. From the set of its successors a new current node has to be chosen. This procedure is repeated until an end node containing the documentation of a method or program is reached.

Complementary to this stepwise guidance, which the user can follow even if he does not know the terms in which to describe his problem, there exists a direct search which allows to enter several keywords, to describe that problem. The system then automatically extracts the paths through the network, connecting the corresponding nodes. If there is more than one method found, decision criteria are displayed, and the user can make his selection. This direct search is suitable for the application specialist, who can describe his problem correctly, but does not know the method and program for its solution.

Before the search for methods can be invoked, the respective information network has to be constructed and fed into the system. The structuring of an application area into an information network is a very important task because the efficiency of the method search highly depends on the quality of the network. It has to be performed by the application expert because only he has the knowledge necessary to break down a general application area into information elements (network nodes), to establish links (network arcs) between these elements and to point out relationships between the elements established and the methods identified. Input of the network structure and the network information is also done interactively with the GAG-System.

## 3. DATA DICTIONARY

### 3.1. Definition, Justification

Retrieval and housekeeping of data is as tedious as finding the proper evaluation program. Therefore, it seems worthwhile to extend the system by a data dictionary component. A data dictionary is the collection of all information known about data. It may contain:

1. Information independent from the physical storage, e.g. meaning and source of data, relationships to other data, relationships to functions. This type of information is intended for the enduser who has to evaluate the data. Therefore it consists mainly of unformatted explanatory text.
2. Information related to data storage, e.g. storage device, file structure, coding. Since this type of information is needed by system functions, e.g. to select the proper functions for data access, conversion, or translation, it consists of formatted data or at least of semi-formal information to be transformed into strongly formatted data.

Current data base systems lack such information, in particular the representation independent part. Therefore, the addition of such a data dictionary might provide a bridge between the enduser and the DB system. Thus, the data dictionary helps to identify the data semantically before the actual values are retrieved with a query language.

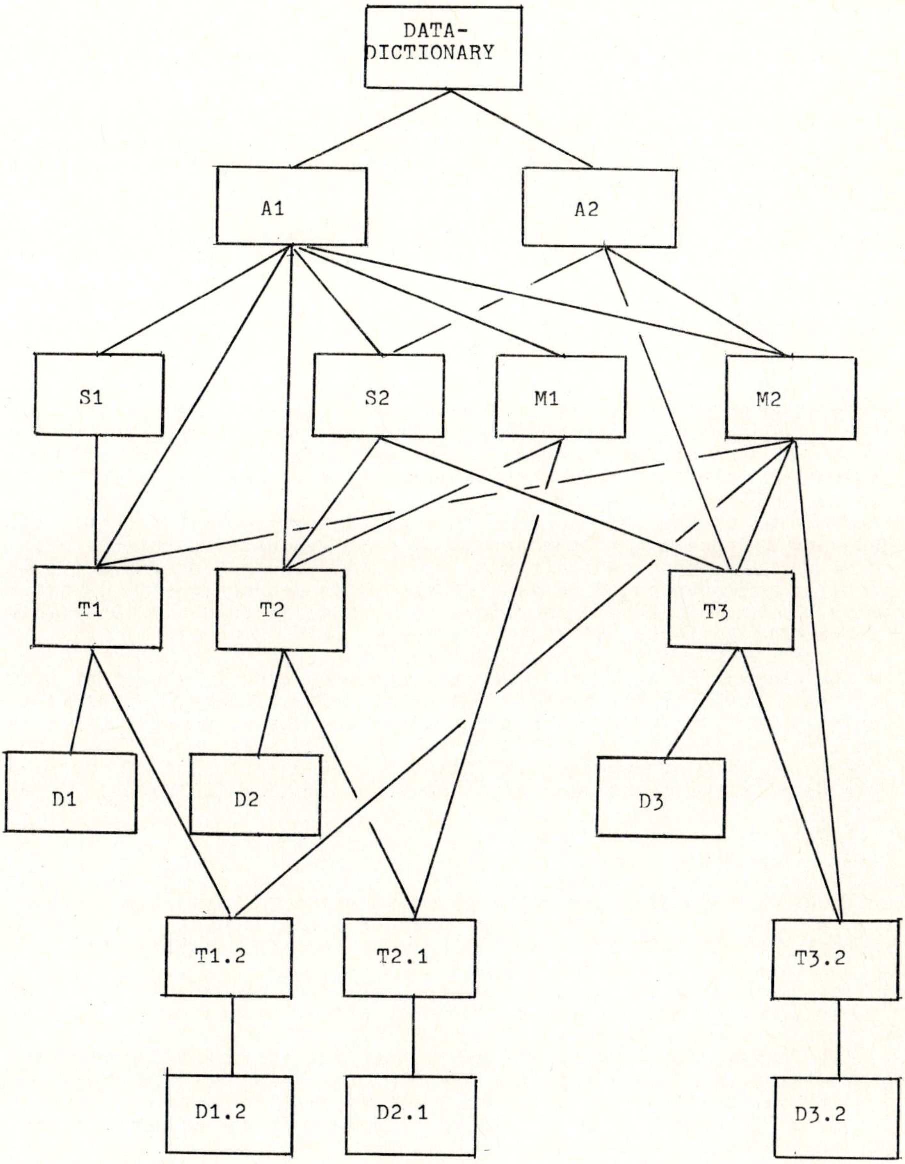


A : Application S : Data-Source D : Data-Directory
M : Method T : Data-Type

Fig. 2: General Example of a Data Dictionary Network.

## 3.2. Network Approach

The data dictionary component is built and accessed for retrieval by the same functions which are used for the methods dictionary.

Descriptions of data elements (files, records, relations, columns, tuples, segments) can be considered as information elements (nodes) in an information network. Common attributes of different elements are described once and linked to the elements by an arc in the network.

In the network approach data elements can be connected concurrently according to different schemata : a source node may refer to all data of the respective source, a node describing an evaluation method refers to all data suitable for that evaluation or to all data generated by its application.

For a general example, consider figure 2 where the highest classification is according to different application fields. At the next level , one grouping corresponds to different data sources, e.g. the result of two different measurement devices, another to different evaluation methods. Then documentation of the data of source S2 is further subdivided into two groups. From every data type description there is an arc to the corresponding data directory of the original data and another arc to the description of evaluated data. The method M1 is connected to data types T2 and T2.1 standing for the original and the evaluated data. Of course this network design is arbitrary. It is left to the application specialist to design that view of the data he wants to see.

The significance of the network approach lies in the fact that this structure is not merely a logical view of data, - described formally for system and system administrator use -, the structure is realized by nodes of textual information, and arcs, which lead from the description of more general facts to the description of details. This description can be accessed and understood by all users.

## 3.3. Consistency Problems

To achieve consistency between data descriptions in the dictionary, as far as formal parameters are concerned, and the actual parameters for data storage, the following rules are established:

1. The data dictionary functions for creation and modification of information are used to enter descriptions of new data, i.e. as a high level data definition tool.
2. The formal data description parameters are automatically extracted from the data description containing unformatted explanatory text as well as strongly formatted information.
3. System functions to write and read data make use of these formal parameters.
4. System functions can create new data only if corresponding data descriptions are available. (They can create new files, but only of a file type already described). Then, the functions also must establish the links from the description to the data, or make entries in directories, which already exist.
5. Modifications of data descriptions which change formal parameters are only allowed if no existing data are referred to by that description. Otherwise a new data description is generated or the modification is rejected.

## 4. EXECUTION OF METHODS

The methods dictionary described in section 2 assists the user in identifying the appropriate method to solve a given application problem. Once a method is found, it is desirable to be able to apply this method without being forced to change the environment of the methods dictionary, i.e. to switch to another system. Sometimes it is necessary to apply a method-1 during a method search session to get decision support for the discrimination between a method-2 and a method-3 (e.g.: the result of a statistical method which tests data on normal distribution must be known before the t-test for the comparison of meanvalues can be chosen).

Thus, it is obvious that the method search by means of a method dictionary has to be extended by a feature for the immediate execution of identified methods or programs.

To make immediate execution possible also for the problem solver without DP-knowledge, execution is designed as a system triggered facility: The user is prompted for entering the necessary input values, and the program is executed automatically by the system.

### 4.1. Program Documentation

The basic information for the system invoked program execution is the program documentation contained in the method dictionary. It is accessed via the respective 'program-node' or more exactly 'program-document-node' which is the successor node of a 'method-node'. The program documentation is set up by the program developer · or another authorized person who is prompted by the GAG-System with characteristic keywords such as PROGRAM-NAME, USE, ARGUMENT, REMARKS, LANGUAGE, TYPE. The prompting facility is introduced to guarantee a standardized documentation which in turn is a prerequisite for a sytem triggered program execution.

The program documentation contains two types of information :

1. Unformatted data for verbal explanations of the program or parts of it such as PURPOSE of the program or EXPLANATION of the meaning of parameters ( see figure 3 for an example ).
2. Formatted information which is absolutely mandatory for the program execution such as USE, UPPER INDICES, TYPE, CONSTRAINTS ( see figure 3 for an example ).

A serious problem is the consistency between program-documentation and program-code. In the present version of the GAG-System the program-documentation is entered manually without automatic extraction of information from the program code. It is felt, however, that the interdependence between documentation and code should be more integrated in the GAG-System such that the formal parts of the documentation are directly derived from the code itself and only the semantic explanation has to be added manually. In addition, it should be made sure that relevant changes in program code invoke automatic update of the documentation. As a prerequisite the program code must be accessible by the GAG-System.

```
* REG12 *
PROGRAM-NAME: REG12
PURPOSE: LINEAR REGRESSION FOR TWO VARIABLES
         INCL. STATISTICAL SIGNIFICANCE TEST FOR THE
         REGRESSION-COEFFICIENT
LANGUAGE: APL
USE: R← Y REG12 X
RIGHT ARGUMENT: X
   TYPE (CHAR,REAL,INT,BOOL): REAL
   UPPER INDICES: *
   EXPLANATION: VALUES OF THE INDEPENDENT VARIABLE
                STORED AS A VECTOR
LEFT ARGUMENT: Y
   TYPE (CHAR,REAL,INT,BOOL): REAL
   UPPER INDICES: *
   EXPLANATION: VALUES OF THE DEPENDENT VARIABLE
                STORED AS A VECTOR
EXPLICIT RESULT: R
   TYPE (CHAR,REAL,INT,BOOL): REAL
   UPPER INDICES: 5
   EXPLANATION: R[1]  REGRESSION-COEFFICIENT OF THE LINE
                      Y = R[1]×X + R[2]
                R[2]  COEFFICIENT OF THE LINE
                      Y = R[1]×X + R[2]
                R[3]  T-VALUE FOR SIGNIFICANCE-TEST (T-TEST)
                      RELATED TO R[1]
                R[4]  NUMBER OF DEGREES OF FREEDOM (T-TEST)
                R[5]  ERROR-PROBABILITY
GLOBAL VARIABLE: TTAB
   TYPE (CHAR,REAL,INT,BOOL): REAL
   UPPER INDICES: 10 3
   READ-WRITE (R,W,RW): R
   EXPLANATION: T-TABLE FOR UP TO 10 DEGREES OF FREEDOM
                AND ERROR-PROBABILITIES .05 .01 .001
CONSTRAINTS: (ρX)=(ρY)
AVAILABLE AT: WS MTB
DATE (DDMMYY): 10. 6.76
AUTHOR: ERBE/H
```

Fig. 3: Example of a Program Documentation (linear regression).

```
EXEC LIN.REGRESSION

PARAMETER-INPUT :
X ← ?
   EXPLANATION: VALUES OF THE INDEPENDENT VARIABLE
                STORED AS A VECTOR
X ← 1 2 3 4 5 6 7 8 9 10
Y ← ?
   EXPLANATION: VALUES OF THE DEPENDENT VARIABLE
                STORED AS A VECTOR
Y ← 3 2 4 5 4 7 3 4 9
(ρX)=(ρY)   : CONSTRAINT NOT FULFILLED !

PARAMETER-INPUT :
X ←
Y ← Y,11.2

RESULT :
R ←         0.726        1.227        3.177        8.000        0.050
?
   EXPLANATION: R[1]  REGRESSION-COEFFICIENT OF THE LINE
                      Y = R[1]×X + R[2]
                R[2]  COEFFICIENT OF THE LINE
                      Y = R[1]×X + R[2]
                R[3]  T-VALUE FOR SIGNIFICANCE-TEST (T-TEST)
                      RELATED TO R[1]
                R[4]  NUMBER OF DEGREES OF FREEDOM (T-TEST)
                R[5]  ERROR-PROBABILITY
EXEC LIN.REGRESSION

PARAMETER-INPUT :
X ← ι10
Y ← YVALUE
YVALUE : VARIABLE/FILE NOT DEFINED !
Y ← YVALUES

RESULT :
R ←         0.779        11.267       4.815        8.000        0.010

YVALUES
10.1 12.2 15.5 14.3 15.9 18.1 16.7 15.9 18.9 17.9
```

Fig. 4: Two Examples of Execution of Linear Regression (user input underscored).

### 4.2. Dialogue

The program independent execution facility of the GAG-System embeds every application program in a dialogue environment without modification of the program itself. Program specific characteristics are considered only at execution time when the documentation is used for prompting and checking the user's input (see figure 4 for examples).

When, after a successful method search, the interactive execution facility is invoked, the user is prompted for the input values. Program parameters can be entered in three different ways:

1. by keying in the values,
2. by entering the names of variables to which values were assigned before, or valid APL expressions of these variables,
3. by the input of a filename invoking standardized I/O-functions accessing the respective files by means of the data dictionary discussed in section 3.

Once the data are entered, they are checked against the information from the program documentation. If there are contradictions of data types, data dimensions or additional constraints of variables or between variables, the entered data are rejected and the input of new data is prompted. If the data are accepted, the program is executed and the results are displayed and stored.

By entering a '?' the user is offered a display of semantic information about selected input or/and output variables.

## 5. SYSTEM GUIDANCE

### 5.1. General Remarks

The information about the use of a special data retrieval and processing system can also be structured as an information network and fed into this guidance system. Then the network can be used instead of a printed user's manual with several advantages:

1. The newcomer can be offered a systematic walk through the complete set of instructions and rules. The information is stored at one place and not scattered over several binders.
2. The user who wants one specific information can be served quickly, either by following a special path through the network, or by addressing directly the point in question.
3. If the guidance system is connected to the system described by it, it may be used as a HELP-feature for the latter one.
4. The structure and the content of the guidance system can easily be updated in case of changes of the system explained. There is no need to print new user manuals or to replace numerous sections in old ones.

This application guidance may best be illustrated by an example, given in the next section, which is a spooled terminal protocol. The concept, the rules for use, and the system features are explained for the GAG-System by GAGS itself.

The descriptions of the features are connected to each other in the same network structure as the features are linked when GAGS is used.

The use of this GAGS-description is invoked automatically when the first question at the start: 'DO YOU KNOW HOW TO USE THIS SYSTEM?' is answered with 'NO'. It can also be accessed by selecting the item GAGS-DESCRIPTION as start node. Thereafter, the further use is decribed extensively by GAGS itself.

## 5.2. Example

Note: For the convenience of the reader, the user input in the following protocol is marked by a preceding '+'.

```
+START
DO YOU KNOW HOW TO USE THIS SYSTEM?
+NO
 THE CURRENT NODE IS:  742 GAGS-DESCRIPTION

 " GAGS-DESCRIPTION "

    HERE THE CONCEPT, THE USAGE RULES, THE SYSTEM FEATURES,

 AND THE FILES FOR 'GAGS' ARE DESCRIBED.

    TO GET MORE INFORMATION, SELECT ONE OF THE ITEMS OF THE

 FOLLOWING LIST BY ENTERING SIMPLY 1, 2, 3, OR 4.

 SELECT FROM THE SUCCESSORS (?=HELP/' '=ESCAPE/S=STATUS):

    1  743 CONCEPTS

    2  744 USAGE-RULES

    3  745 FEATURES

    4  746 GAGS-FILES

    5  756 END-GUIDANCE

+1
 THE CURRENT NODE IS:  743 CONCEPTS

 " CONCEPTS "

    THE MOST IMPORTANT FACT IN 'GAGS' IS THAT THE INFORMA-

 TION IS DIVIDED IN SMALL PARTS. THESE PARTS ARE CONNECTED TO

 EACH OTHER, ACCORDING TO THEIR SEMANTICS, IN A NETWORK LIKE

 STRUCTURE.  THEREFORE THE INFORMATION PARTS ARE CALLED

 NODES, THE LINKS ARE CALLED ARCS.

    .....
    TO PROCEED, SELECT ONE OF THE ITEMS OF THE FOLLOWING

 LIST BY ENTERING 1, 2, OR 3.
```

```
SELECT FROM THE SUCCESSORS (?=HELP/' '=ESCAPE/S=STATUS):

   1  744 USAGE-RULES

   2  745 FEATURES

   3  746 GAGS-FILES

   4  756 END-GUIDANCE

+1
THE CURRENT NODE IS:  744 USAGE-RULES

" USAGE-RULES "

   HERE, THE IMPORTANT RULES FOR THE BEGINNER ARE GIVEN.
FURTHER DETAILS ARE FOUND IN THE NODES 'DIALOGUE-MODES' AND
'HELP-FUNCTION'.

   .....

SELECT FROM THE SUCCESSORS (?=HELP/' '=ESCAPE/S=STATUS):

   1  747 DIALOGUE-MODES

   2  748 HELP-FUNCTION

   3  745 FEATURES

   4  746 GAGS-FILES

   5  756 END-GUIDANCE

+1
THE CURRENT NODE IS:  747 DIALOGUE-MODES

" DIALOGUE-MODES "

   THERE ARE TWO DIALOGUE MODES CONCURRENTLY AVAILABLE:
PROMPT-MODE AND  COMMAND-MODE.

   THE HINTS, GIVEN IN 'USAGE-RULES' RELATE TO THE PROMPT-
MODE WHERE, IN ADDITION, TWO DIFFERENT LENGTHS OF GAGS-
MESSAGES ARE OFFERED. MOREOVER, DIFFERENT NATURAL LANGUAGES
ARE AVAILABLE, AT PRESENT ENGLISH AND GERMAN.

   FURTHER DETAILS ARE FOUND IN THE NODES 'PROMPT-MODE',
'COMMAND-MODE', AND IST SUCCESSORS.
   .....
```

Note: At this point, the protocol is cut off.

## 6. EXPERIMENTAL SYSTEM

Based on the ideas outlined in the chapters 2 to 5, a dialogue system has been implemented using APL/CMS /5/. The choice of APL/CMS as implementation language offers great advantages for the implementor due to its nature as a dialogue system and its support for implementing, debugging, and modifying functions, adding new functions, and thereby extending the system. It does not influence the user's view of the system, in effect, he is not aware of APL.

The dialogue system is selfexplanatory. Optionally, a description of system usage is given at start time (see also chapter 5). Further information may be requested via a help function entering '?' whenever user input is expected. The help option offers explanations for system or application oriented keywords unknown to the user. If the user enters keywords that do not match a keyword for which an explanation is stored, a search for similar keywords is performed /4/. In case that no similar keyword is found the keyword entered is stored to permit the data base administrator to add the respective explanation.

There exist two complementary versions for the man machine dialogue: the prompting mode and the command mode /6/. In the prompting mode there is never a need for the user to remember the options which are available. In each state, all possibilities are made visible in a multiple choice menu or by a yes/no question. In the command mode the display of menus and questions is suppressed. The user selects options and answers to anticipated questions by entering commands. In general, a command is the main keyword taken from the dialogue item which it replaces. Only when the user requests prompting by '?' or when he enters an invalid command, the question or menu is displayed. Several commands may be entered in one line. At any time the user can switch between prompting and command mode. Thus, when the casual user develops towards the trained user he can make more efficient use of GAGS.

For the reason of information security, different user classes are introduced. Users with write permission are registered in a directory. Usage of the network construction part of the system is only possible after successful pass-control.

The system is a multi-user system which allows for concurrent retrieval, insertion and update by several users. To provide multi-user access to a consistent version of latest information , all application dependent information which is subject to updates, e.g. the list of node names, the textual node information, and the binary relation representing the network structure, is stored in files outside the APL workspace.

The dialogue system consists of five sets of functions:

1. Search functions for the enduser who wants to retrieve information. In case of method search the search functions are complemented by the method execution part.
2. Build functions used by the application specialist to build the information network and to store the respective information.
3. Modify functions to change the information structure and to update obsolete parts of information.
4. Delete functions to erase nodes and respective information.
5. Comment functions to establish a communication bridge between endusers on the one hand, and network architects, information suppliers , and the system administrator on the other hand.

## 7. SUMMARY

The GAG-System described here helps the user in the problem solving environment in four ways: confronted with a specific problem constellation the enduser who is not a DP-professional is supported to find the appropriate solution method(s), to identify the data to be processed by the identified method(s), to execute the methods and finally he is assisted in the use of information processing systems.

The fundamental information structure for the dialogue oriented guidance of the GAG-System is the information network. Both functions, the use of the information networks for the interactive guidance of the enduser as well as the construction of the networks by the respective application experts are integrated in the GAG-System.

The GAG-System is not tailored to a special application. In principle, every application area for which information-networks can be set up, can be fed into the system.

The GAG-System can be employed by users with different levels of experience in GAGS as well as in the application area. GAGS offers menu type dialogue for the beginner and provides command type dialogue for the advanced user. Application oriented information can be requested in two different modes. The beginner is guided through the information network whereas the advanced user can invoke a more direct search by entering problem describing keywords.

## 8. REFERENCES

1. Brunnstein, K., Schmidt, J.W. (1973). Structuring and Retrieving Information in Computer Based Learning, Int.J.Computer & Information Sciences, No. 2, 89
2. Erbe, R., Walch, G. (1975). An Interactive Guidance System for Method Libraries, IBM Scient. Cent. TR 75.04.001, Heidelberg
3. Erbe, R., Walch, G. (1975). Ein Dialogsystem zur Methodensuche, Lecture Notes in Computer Science, GI-5. Annual Congress, Springer Berlin, Heidelberg, New York
4. Erbe, R., Schek, H.J. (1975). Search with Fuzzy Keywords in a Methods Data Base, IBM Scient. Cent. TR 75.05.003, Heidelberg
5. IBM (1974). APL/CMS User's Manual, Programming RPQ MF2608, IBM File No.S370.22, Order No. SC20.1846
6. Walch, G. (to be published). Dialogue Programming with Easy Transition from Prompting- to Command-Mode, IBM Scient. Cent. TR, Heidelberg
7. Wexler, J.D. (1970). Information Networks in Generative Computer Aided Instruction, IEEE MMS No. 11, 181

*Systems for Large Data Bases, P.C. Lockemann and E.J. Neuhold, (eds.)*
*North-Holland Publishing Company, 1976*

# MERLIN

# DESIGN OF A NATIONAL BIBLIOGRAPHIC DATABASE

P.L. Noerr and M.C. White
Bibliographic Services Division
The British Library, London

This paper describes MERLIN, the British Library's national bibliographic information retrieval system. It describes the functions performed by the system and the users for whom it is intended. In particular it outlines the main problems associated with bibliographic data for a national library.

The logical design of the database is discussed with particular reference to the space economy necessary for a database of 3 million items. A highly shared structure, which allows flexibility as well as economy of storage, is proposed. Methods of access, authority handling and creation of private views are given.

## INTRODUCTION

The British Library is a government funded body set up in 1974 to provide information services to the whole United Kingdom. The range of services cover the following areas:-

a) Reference facilities; the Reference Division currently has some 10 million books and periodicals available for reference, including all material deposited by publishers under the copyright legislation.

b) Lending facilities; the Lending Division holds a large collection of material of current interest to lend to any library to satisfy a short term need for any item not in their own stocks. Requests for material which the Lending Division does not have in its own stocks are often satisfied by referring the request to a library which does have the necessary material.

c) Bibliographic services; the Bibliographic Services Division offers a range of automated services to libraries, including the British Library's Reference and Lending Divisions, and other information users such as universities and industries. The main services provided are:-

   i) the British National Bibliography (BNB); this is a weekly bibliography of all books published in the United Kingdom, and is computer produced using phototypesetting techniques.

   ii) exchange tapes; these are weekly produced magnetic tapes containing the records published in the BNB. The records are in an international standard format, the MARC (MAchine Readable Catalogue) format. MARC records are received by the British Library from other international sources such as the Library of Congress, and distributed as exchange tapes.

The exchange tapes are used by libraries to produce local catalogues or operate Selective Dissemination of Information (SDI) services.

iii) selective record services; records from the above sources can be selected by ISBN (International Standard Book Number) on demand, rather than being supplied weekly in bulk.

iv) catalogue production service; this increasingly popular service produces catalogues, for any subscribing library, of all books and other items that it acquires. A catalogue is a list of books, in a prescribed order, containing bibliographic information (author, title, subject etc) and local information (shelf location, acquisition number etc) for each book. The bibliographic information can largely be taken from records produced by the British Library, or Library of Congress etc, whereas the local information must be input by the local library. Most libraries have three separately defined catalogues for the same collection of material. This is to allow for a number of different methods of finding the same book. Catalogues are produced on microfiche, microfilm, printed on paper or cards or phototypeset.

v) regional lending lists; many UK libraries subscribe to one of nine regional library bureaux. Each bureau is provided by the BL with a microfilmed list of all books held by each subscribing library in its region. This greatly enhances the capability of each library to borrow books from neighbouring libraries.

The Computer Services Office is currently developing a new system called MERLIN (MachinE Readable Library InformatioN) to integrate the services of the Bibliographic Services Division. MERLIN will provide the full range of services outlined above and, in addition, will provide an on-line information retrieval service.

The on-line service will enhance, and to some extent supplant, the existing range of services, by enabling users to consult the MERLIN database directly about books in their own or other libraries' stocks. Thus the process of satisfying an enquirer's needs, borrowing from other libraries and purchasing books will all be facilitated, saving time and money.

The cataloguing by a library of its acquisitions is greatly simplified if a book has already been described, or at least the author and subject information is immediately available. This latter information is used for authority checking, which is required by the Anglo-American Cataloguing Rules. These require, for example, that an individual author is described accurately and sufficiently fully to distinguish him from any other person, by adding forenames, dates of birth etc as necessary. Authority handling is described later in this paper in some detail.

It has been decided to implement MERLIN with a single integrated database as this seems to confer two real advantages over the previous method, which was oriented towards user files. The advantages have been briefly mentioned above as being

a) minimisation of input duplication, with the consequent cost saving and better chance of obtaining data integrity.

b) the whole database is available to any user at any time.

THE NATURE OF THE DATA

The MERLIN database will hold bibliographic descriptions of a large variety of material types, including books, periodicals, films, sound recordings, videotapes, educational kits, etc; the collections or series to which any of these belong; and the volumes, chapters, reels, etc, which constitute any of them. For brevity, and because they do occur most frequently in libraries, we will refer to all of these bibliographic entities as 'books' for the rest of this paper.

In 1978 there will be descriptions of 1.1 million books catalogued by the British Library, and 0.8 million catalogued by the Library of Congress. An annual growth rate of 130,000 records from these sources produces a volume of 2.16 million in 1980. By this date it is expected that 44 external libraries and other users will be contributing to the system, and as each has an average of 200,000 books in their own holdings this adds 8.8 million making a total of 11 million.

A typical MARC description requires 600 characters per book, thus the actual volume of data will be approximately 6,600 MBytes or $5.3 \times 10^{10}$ bits.

This would be the size of the database if all the data were to be stored redundantly, without any sort of indexing for access. This indexing would add something between 50% and 100% to the size.

There are over 200 internationally recognised distinctive descriptive elements (e.g. author, editor, title, classification, publisher, etc) that can be used in the description of a book. In practice only 20 of these are used, on average, to describe any one book. However, no one element is necessarily always present, so there can be no primary key. Equally all fields may be present more than once in any one description, even, unfortunately, the unique international standard book number (ISBN) supposedly assigned to every book. Because of this variation it is necessary to allow that every field can be used as an access key.

Any particular field may vary in the size of its contents over quite a wide range (e.g. title: i) Hamlet, ii) Annual Review of Information Science and Technology).

The previously quoted volume (11 million books at 1980) refers to individual libraries' views of books, and in reality represents 2.75 million different publications. It is, however, essential that the individual views of the 2.75 million books be maintained, as each library may have its own conventions for, say, classifying books, and will, in any case, want to record wholly private information such as the shelf position of the book, the order number, number of copies and so on.

Of the 20 fields used to describe the book it is expected that, on average, 15 of them will be common to the views of all users (librarians can usually agree on the form of author names, titles, etc). It thus becomes evident that the problem becomes one of having several private views of a set of shared book descriptions.

MERLIN makes use of this fact and will store 2.75 million common book descriptions each with one or more user specific private views. The common, or public, part of the description is in fact the private view of the most 'trusted' of the users who have a view of that book. 'Trustedness' is practically achieved by holding a list of all data contributors and grading them according to such things as error rate, the subject specialists available as indexers, and the policy of the particular user with regard to the standards and conventions in use. This is purely a measure of how useful the information is for other users of the system.

Each user views a book description on the database through a virtual record. This will show him the public view of that book, modified and extended by any changes which he has made to the public view. If he has made no changes then he will see the unchanged public view.

## DATA MODEL

The nature of bibliographic information clearly presents a number of difficulties. The major ones outlined so far are:-

a) variability of field size

b) variability of field occurance

c) absence of a candidate key for book records

Taking into account all of the previously outlined data characteristics, some of the possible logical record structures for the database will be examined. These are shown diagrammatically in Fig.1.

The best established conventional record technique is shown in diagram 1 (Fig.1). In this each possible field has a fixed position and size reserved for it. This clearly gives rise to both wastage of space and a danger of truncation of the larger fields. Most existing database management systems use a data model of this sort, for example any system based on the CODASYL proposals will.

The variability of field occurance can be overcome by identifying each field with a 'tag' as in diagram 2 (Fig.1), but to fully overcome the problems, each field should be allowed to vary in length as in diagram 3 (Fig.1). This is essentially the MARC record format. The 'tag' is used to identify a field and a delimiter is used to end it. A given tag can occur more than once and thus has to be 'addressed' by the tag plus an occurance count (e.g. 100/2 - the second author(100) field).

The MARC record format is used in MERLIN as the input/output format. The user stores and retrieves records to and from the database in virtual records in this format.

This is still not the ideal storage vehicle as a given field may be common to more than one book (e.g. William Shakespeare wrote many books). This is important for two reasons:-

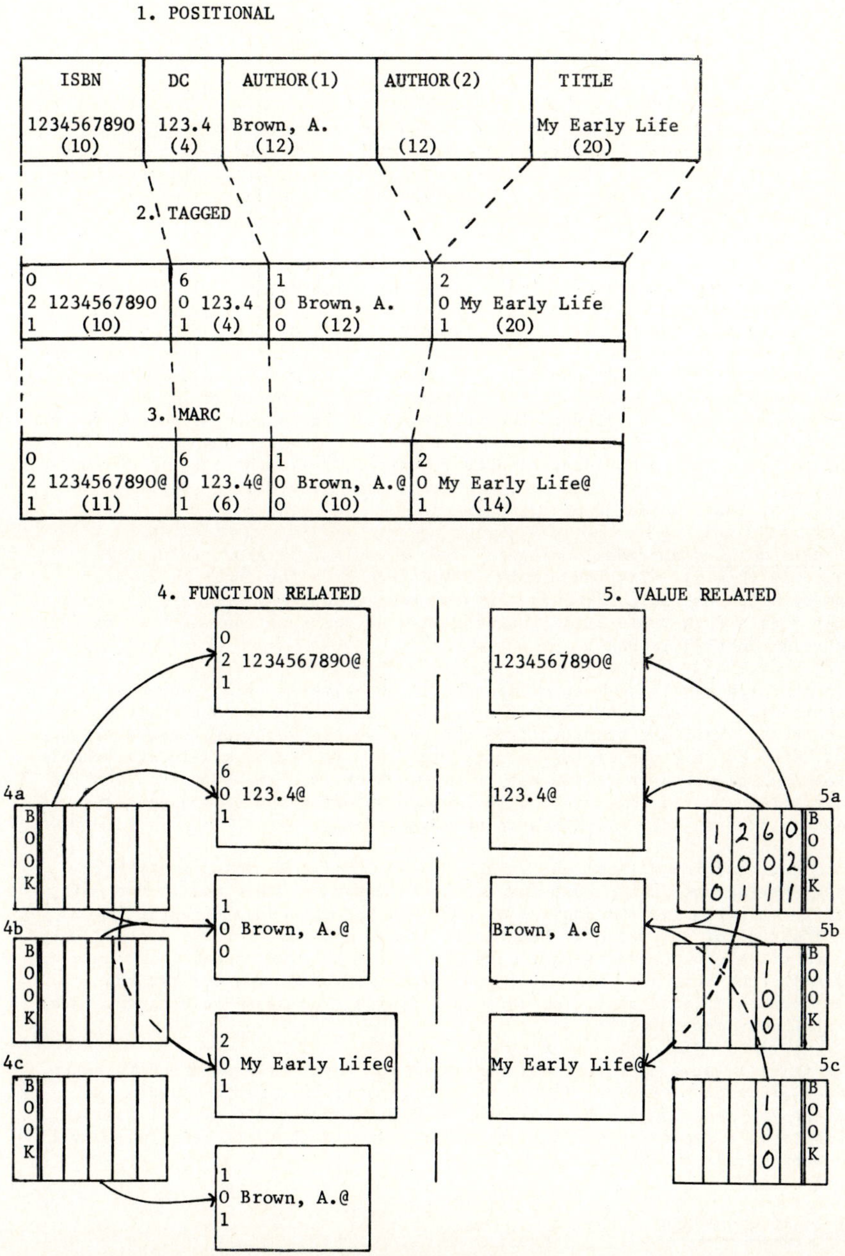


FIG. 1: LOGICAL DATA REPRESENTATIONS

1. Space can be saved by two books sharing the same piece of data.

2. A descriptive field may be a sensible entity in its own right (e.g. William Shakespeare is a real person, represented by a unique set of details such as name and birth and death dates etc). The treatment of William Shakespeare in this fashion as an independent entity is an example of authority handling.

Diagram 4a (Fig.1) shows a function related approach to tackling this problem. In this the book record contains nothing but pointers to field records. Each field record contains a tag and the field contents or value. Thus when a new book by the same author is introduced (4b) there are two books sharing a common author field. Diagram 4c demonstrates the main shortcoming of the function related approach. It shows a book which has as editor the same person as the author of the previous books. Thus there is not entity independence and the value of the entity could not be changed just once for all occurances e.g. Winston Churchill would have to be changed to Sir Winston Churchill for all occurances as author, editor, collector etc. Also important is that space has been used over and above that necessary to indicate the different function being performed.

A value related approach, using the same examples, is shown in diagrams 5a to 5c (Fig.1). The fundamental difference from the function related approach is that each element is now stored without any tagging, it is now stored as a data value quite independently of the function which it performs in relation to any books.

The function tags have been stripped off the value as being unnecessarily restrictive. These functions must still be indicated in some fashion for each book. Thus the pointers from the book to the value are tagged to indicate the function of the value in relation to the book. In the example the same value serves as the author of two books and the editor of a third. This more correctly mirrors the real state of affairs as the author and editor are, in reality, the same person.

Both the function related and value related approaches allow a distinct space saving over the previously mentioned methods. This is, in the main, due to allowing for the sharing of data and the consequent flexibility as to the size of the values. Between these two methods there is a complicated space trade-off depending on the ratios of tag to data sizes, the occurance of different tags for one value, and the number of fields per record. It has been calculated that, for this application, the value related approach is the more economical.

The value related approach corresponds to the three dimensional data space model proposed by Bachman (1973) where the entity-attribute-measure is matched by book-tag-value. This approach meets all the previously raised objectives for storing bibliographic data, and is the data model which will be adopted for the MERLIN database.

## DATABASE STRUCTURE

So far it has been shown that two types of record exist; one to represent a book, the other a value. The book record uses tagged pointers to identify a value and to indicate its function. Similarly a value record uses tagged pointers to identify its functions in relation to books. Tagging a relation in both directions optimises retrieval, as it is never necessary to follow a link, only to discover that the linked-to record is not wanted.

For these links pointer lists (or arrays) are used rather than chains. This avoids the necessity of having to tag, or physically reserve, the continuation pointers for the chain. Lists have the even bigger advantage that retrieval for searches which use Boolean manipulation of the results can be done without having to acccss the records.

The database record consists of two types of elements; lists, and values. An identifier distinguishes the two types of element so that as many as necessary of each type may be combined within a given entity record.

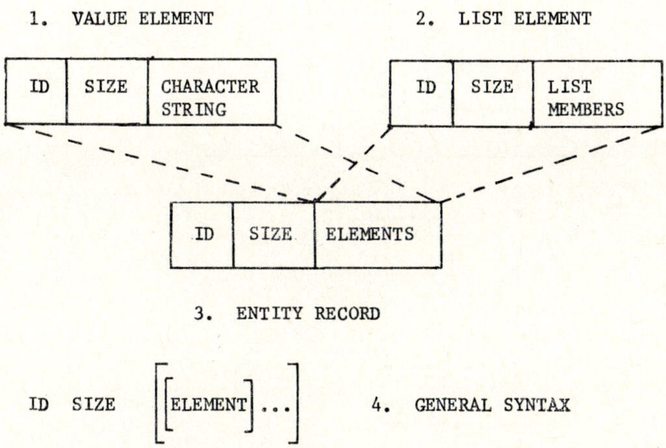


FIG.2: DATABASE ITEM SYNTAX

Diagram 1 (Fig.2) shows the representation used for a value element. The identifier labels the subsequent information as pertaining to a value. This is followed by a self-defining size indicator which gives the size of the immediately following character string.

Diagram 2 (Fig.2) shows the representation used for a list element. In this case the identifier labels the subsequent information as belonging to a list, states the nature of the list members, and includes a self-defining tag which identifies the function represented by the list. The size of each list member is inherent in its nature and thus the number of members of a list is calculable from the list size.

The consistency of representation of both value and list elements is obvious and diagram 4 (Fig.2) shows the general syntactic representation of this. This is a basic three part scheme for representing units of the database and consists of an identifier, a size, and the elements.

This general syntax also applies to the entity record. This situation is shown in diagram 3 (Fig.2). The identifier indicates a record and the entity type (value, book, etc). In the latter case, a tag indicates the bibliographic category of the record (book, article, series, etc). This is followed by a size indicator which gives the total size of the record. The elements of the record can be either lists or values, thus nesting the syntactic description of the database structure to a depth of two.

ENTITIES AND RELATIONS

Thus far only book and value entities have been considered, as they collectively are the whole information content of the database. Fig.3 gives a complete entity diagram of the database and introduces additional entities and relations.

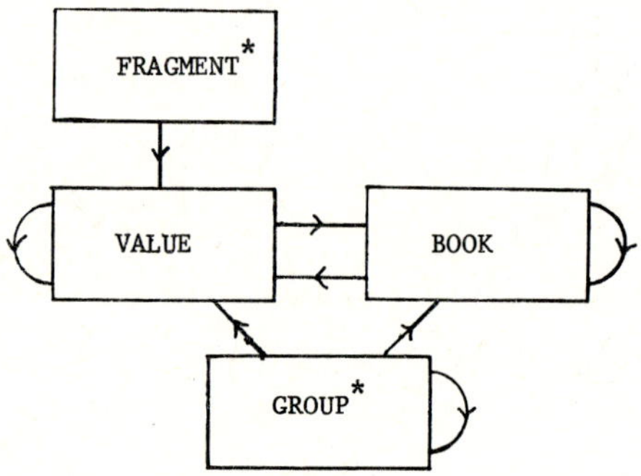


FIG.3: ENTITY DIAGRAM

a) Fragment entities; these provide direct access to the value entities, by their contents. Each value entity contains a character string (its value)which can be divided into one or more subfields. For example, the value entity 'William Shakespeare' consists of two subfields: 'William' and 'Shakespeare'. These subfields are both useful access points, and thus a fragment record would be created for each. In fact, fragment records are created for all subfields.

   Fragment records thus provide content addressability for all value entities stored on the database, and hence permit retrieval of books by any descriptive element. A fragment record contains a value element (a subfield) and lists. Links from fragments to value entities are not reciprocated. This is because they redundantly repeat value data for efficiency, and are potentially disposable when content addressable mass storage becomes readily available.

b) Group entities; these enable sets of value or book entities to be represented. Each group has a tag, through which it is accessed, identifying the group.

   i) Value entity groups are similar in concept to the domain of the relational data model. They can be ordered on value if desired.

Thus an ordered set of all values used as authors could be created. Range searching, browsing, and mass retrieval by this attribute are thus enabled.

ii) Book entity groups are similar in concept to the relation of the relational data model, they are used mainly to represent groups of books which could not be dynamically created efficiently by searching on value. Only one type of book entity group is created automatically. For each user all books of which he owns a view will be formed into a group. Other groups can be created manually by searching and logically creating the desired set of book records, which then have a group record set up with a pointer to each of them, (e.g. a group of 16th century religious works to which frequent subsequent reference is to be made). These manually created groups are a performance and convenience aid as they can always be dynamically re-created by searching on the values.

iii) Groups of groups can be manually created to construct even larger sets of book or value entities. As with fragments, the links from groups to their members are not reciprocated.

c) Book entities; these, as previusly explained, represent true bibliographic entities, the storage of which is the object of this system. Each entity record is fully self defining; i.e. although no record has a primary key per se, it is identified by having a unique set of attribute/value pairs. A book entity contains no value elements, only lists. These are of two types:-

i) Attributes; an attribute list exists for each attribute of a book. Each list has a tag defining the attribute (e.g. 100 = author), and a pointer to the appropriate value. Additional pointers, qualified by user identification, may exist in the list if any users have a private view of this attribute. This is discussed more fully below.

ii) Entity relations; a given entity may have a part-whole relation with another (e.g. a book may be in a series, a volume may contain chapters - each of these items would be stored as a separate book entity, each with its own attributes). This means that a book entity may be part of an intellectually created bibliographic hierarchy. For each relation that a book entity has, a list pointing to the appropriate entity is created. The list's tag identifies the relation as being either whole-part or part-whole. Horizontal relations can also exist (e.g. where a book is a translation or revision of another), and a further range of tags enables any of these relations to be expressed. (In fact, over 30 horizontal relation types are recognised). All these relations have reciprocals and these are automatically created. As with attribute lists, private views of book entity relations can be established.

d) Value entities; these contain a single value element and one or more lists. These lists are of two types:-

i) Function lists; these reciprocate the attribute lists in the book entity records, and each one is tagged to indicate the nature of the relation (e.g. used as author, used as subject term, etc). These links exist solely for retrieval purposes and enable the selection of books by any of their attributes.

ii) Authority Packet lists; these lists enable values which represent a real entity (e.g. William Shakespeare) to have globally defined relations expressed for them. This effectively enables thesaurus structures to be made. The tag 'alternative spelling' when used between the values 'William Shakespeare' and 'William Shagspear' enables the latter to be referenced from any book which has the former assigned as an attribute.

This technique of handling value records as entities in their own right is known as authority handling, and a particular value record treated in this way with its related value records (if any) constitute an authority packet. In retrieval and update terms, an authority packet is viewed as a virtual record consisting of one or more fields and is merely a special case of the treatment of books. As with other list types private views of authority packet links can be set up. Because authority packets are virtual entities their value can be changed as well as their relations. Thus one change will be reflected in uses right across the database. As only the most 'trusted' users may actually change the public view of data, an attempted value change by a less trusted user will result in the setting up of an altered private copy of the value record itself, pointed to by a special list meaning 'private view of this value'.

## VIRTUAL RECORDS

As mentioned before the virtual record is the users unit of logical storage and retrieval for the database, and is generally displayed in the MARC format. This is particularly true for the user who is an indexer or cataloguer or other bibliographic expert. However for retrieval purposes it is often necessary to perform both data conversion and format changes to arrive at a suitable display for a non-specialist.

The user supplies a virtual record profile which defines the attributes that he is interested in for a given application. This profile also indicates the scope of the entity hierarchy to be considered and any data conversions to be performed.

Retrieval is initiated by a search function which results in a set of book records being identified, which satisfy the search criteria. Each book record is then considered as the root of a tree of related book and value entities to construct the desired virtual records. This logical tree (Fig.4) is limited by the following rules:-

i) 'contains' links may be followed as far as desired. (Fig.4: A contains D contains E & F etc).

ii) 'contained in' links are treated similarly. (Fig.4: A contained in B contained in C etc).

iii) horizontal links may be followed only one step.
(Fig.4: A translated from I; has supplement J)

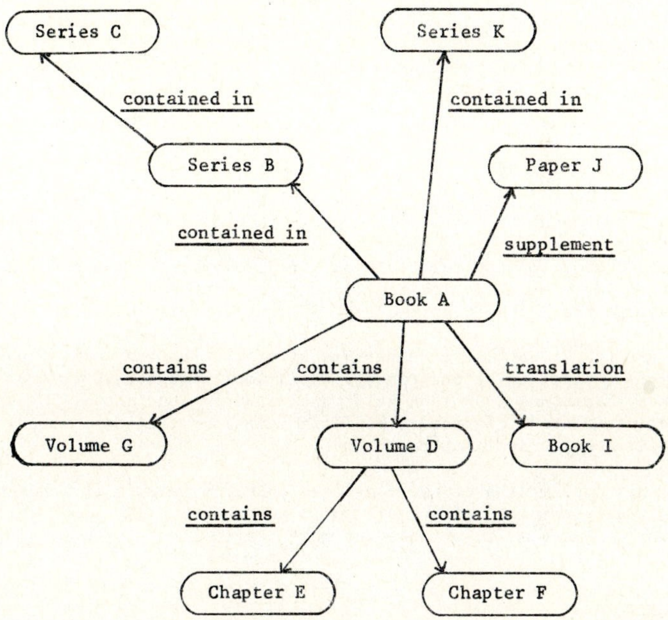


FIG. 4: VIRTUAL RECORD CONSTRUCTION

Attribute tags are prefixed by a relation tag where the values are attributes of a related entity rather than the root entity.

No mention has yet been made of private views on output. It should be evident, however, that as each relation is checked for inclusion in a virtual record its list will be scanned to determine if the user has a private view of the relation. If he has this will over-ride the public view. Four basic types of private view exist, they are:-

i) private attributes of a book entity; additional attributes, nullified attributes, attributes with a different value.

ii) private book entity relations; additional, nullified or changed relations.

iii) private authority packet value; changed value of an authority value entity.

iv) private authority packet relations; additional, nullified or changed value entity relations for this user's authority packets.

Each user believes that he has unlimited access to all of the database, and is allowed to change or add to any part of it. Private views are to protect all such users from the effects of other user's changes whilst still allowing a high degree of data sharing. Each user always sees his own private view of the data, which is the public view as modified by him.

## CONCLUSION

The objective of the MERLIN system design has been to produce a fully structured database which will support information retrieval efficiently. The problems inherent in the data; its variability, lack of candidate key, and many to many relations had to be overcome. The best approach was considered to be the value related and this appears to allow the system to bridge the gap between the DBM and IR requirements successfully.

Its use in this application derives directly from the work of one of the authors (Noerr, to be published). This work itself derives from earlier work by Farradane (1966) on Relational Indexing and shows that the principle of value related information handling (concept-relation-concept) has a totally general application.

For this application we are convinced that not only is the chosen solution practically the most efficient, but also theoretically sound. It would appear to be equally suitable for more conventional database applications.

## REFERENCES

Bachman C.W. (1973), Data Space Mapped Into Three Dimensions. In: Infotech State of the Art no. 15 - Data Base Management, 431-453.

Farradane J.E.L. et al (1966), Report on Information Retrieval by Relational Indexing. The City University, London.

Noerr P.L. (to be published), Information, Structure, Network, Retrieval. In: Informatics 4. Proceedings of a conference held by the Aslib Co-ordinate Indexing Group on 5-7 April 1976 at Lancaster University, England.

# AUTHOR INDEX

Corrigenda

p.6, 11th line from below: delete [ANSI]

p.17, upper part of the figure:
ALGORITHM SPECIFIED BY APPLICATION ADMINISTRATOR

p.74, 18th line from below:
invoking P1 through P7 is estimated to be 25%, 25%, 20%, 10%, 10%, 5%, and 5% respectively.

p.112, 6th line from below:
(iii) While checking through the A tuples in (ii) we . . . .

p.116, 3rd line from below:
Su, S.Y.W., Copland, G.P. and Lipovski, G.P. (1973). . . .

p.123, 8th line from above:
.... By application of string switching (and skipping) the ....

p.127, 7th line from above: ..... is shown in the L-string Flight;....

p.136, concerning underline:
1st line from above:
PASSENGERS (PLANE ID, SEAT ID, PASS NAME, ADDRESS)

3rd line from above:
PASS (PASS NAME, ADDRESS, SEAT ID, PLANE ID, TYPE, LOC,

6th line from above:
LOCATION(LOC)

p.137, fig.14, 9th line from above:

SEGM NAME=PASSENGER, BYTES=29, FREQ=50,PTR=H,PARENT=AIRPLANE

p.150, fig.2, alter the 4 last lines to:

```
PROJ1(D1#,DNAME1,DMGR1,E1#,ENAME1,SEX1,SCH1)<----SELECT(D#,DNAME,DMGR,E#, ENAME,
                                                  SEX,SCHOOL FROM IEMP:IEMP.PROJ=1)
PROJ2(D2#,DNAME2,DMGR2,E2#,ENAME2,SEX2,SCH2)<----SELECT(D#,DNAME,DMGR,E#,ENAME,
                                                  SEX,SCHOOL FROM IEMP:IEMP.PROJ=2)
PROJ3(D3#,DNAME3,DMGR3,E3#,ENAME3,SEX3,SCH3)<----SELECT(D#,DNAME,DMGR,E#,ENAME,
                                                  SEX,SCHOOL FROM IEMP:IEMP.PROJ=3)
DEPTBUDG(DEPT#,DNAME,DMGR,BUDGET) <----DEPT(D#,DNAME,DMGR,BUDGT);
```